10 SIMPLE TR
THAT WILL
SET YOU FREE

YOUR

AN OWNER'S MANUAL

FOR A BETTER LIFE

MIND

Dr. Christopher Cortman
Dr. Harold Shinitzky

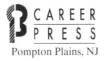

CAREER
PRESS
Pompton Plains, NJ

YOUR MIND: AN OWNER'S MANUAL FOR A BETTER LIFE
EDITED BY KIRSTEN DALLEY
TYPESET BY EILEEN MUNSON
Cover design by Howard Grossman / 12E Design
Printed in the U.S.A.

To order this title, please call toll-free 1-800-CAREER-1 (NJ and Canada: 201-848-0310) to order using VISA or MasterCard, or for further information on books from Career Press.

The Career Press, Inc., 220 West Parkway, Unit 12
Pompton Plains, NJ
www.careerpress.com

Library of Congress Cataloging-in-Publication Data

Cortman, Christopher.
Your mind : an owner's manual for a better life : 10 simple truths that will set you free / by Christopher Cortman and Harold Shinitzky.
p. cm.
Includes index.
ISBN 978-1-60163-080-3
1. Mental health. 2. Emotions. I. Shinitzky, Harold. II. Title.

RA790.C68198 2010
616.89--dc22

2009036388

Acknowledgments

Chris: Thanks to Dr. Jill Scarpellini, for your insights and contributions to the 10 Truths; Stephanie, for your love and unyielding support; Shaina, for voluntary editorial contributions; Peggy and Debby, for clerical excellence; Laurie Rosin, for editorial insights; Principal Candace Millington, for believing in our vision to make the 10 Truths a staple in the schools; and to family and friends, too many to mention by name. Most of all, to 4-year-old Cameron and baby Melina, the loves of my life, who inspire me daily to be the best man I can be.

Harold: Thank you to my family for their lifelong love and support, and to my friends for their encouragement and belief. I'd also like to express my gratitude to my Johns Hopkins University School of Medicine family, Drs. Schretlen, Edwin, and Brandt, and Drs. Adger, Oski, Wilson, and Joffe, for their encyclopedic knowledge, exceptional clinical acumen, and passionate desire to be the best role models anyone could hope for. They set the bar high and expect nothing but the best from those whom they mentor.

Both of us would also like to thank Dottie, for her ongoing reviews; Betsy Steiner, for her vision and partnership; Bruce Wexler, for his editorial expertise; our agent, Pilar Queen, for her support, publishing industry acumen, and belief in the book; and Michael Pye, Adam Schwartz, and all the other great people at Career Press, for turning the manuscript into an even better book.

Lastly, we would like to thank each and every one of our patients and their family members. This book has evolved from our interactions and would not be possible without them. It has been an honor to help make a difference in their lives.

Table of Contents

Introduction

How well do you understand how your mind works?

The odds are you possess a better understanding of how your car works. You probably have a much better sense of how your computer functions. And, if you're like most people, you are more knowledgeable about other parts of your body—for example, you probably know why your knee is chronically sore, or how exercise affects your heart rate.

For a long time, we've depended on therapists to tell us about our minds. To a certain extent that's fine. As psychologists, we've undergone extensive training to help our patients, and we've had more than 40 years of combined clinical experience on a wide range of issues. Perhaps even more important from a communication perspective, both of us have worked in the media, interpreting psychological issues for lay audiences. This is part of what we offer in this book. But there's no reason that people can't also help themselves. In fact, our patients who grasp the principles discussed in this book tend to get better faster than those who don't grasp them.

Even if you're not in therapy, these principles can assist you in all areas of your life. If you understand how your mind works—if you know why you feel inexplicably sad at certain times or why you seem to sabotage certain types of relationships, for example—you can help yourself in many ways, including:

▶ Healing from an emotional trauma in your past.

▶ Learning how to establish and maintain more rewarding relationships.

- ▶ Dealing more effectively with problems at work.

- ▶ Managing and minimizing addictive behaviors.

- ▶ Finding more happiness and meaning in your life.

We made it our mission to research what the key psychological principles are, and then communicate them in a way that would make them useful for readers. To that end, we created our own list of what we thought were the most important ideas about the mind and then talked to other therapists to get their feedback. We also relied on our extensive experience working with patients on a wide range of issues.

The result of our work has been identifying 10 psychological principles—the 10 Truths—you'll find in the following pages. (We decided to call them truths because "principles" sounds too academic and forbidding.) Plus, as you'll discover, these really *are* Truths about how the mind works. An ounce of prevention is worth a pound of cure, and these Truths will protect you from many of the mistakes you currently make because you lack sufficient knowledge about your mind.

The 10 Truths and How You Can Use Them

In a moment, we're going to provide you with a list of the 10 Truths. Before reading them, we want you to understand that this isn't a definitive list by any means. Another psychologist might create a somewhat different set of Truths—20 Truths instead of 10, or the Truths would be worded differently. In addition, these Truths aren't the result of a recent breakthrough study; many therapists are aware of these principles but have just never crystallized them in this form. Still, we believe this is a representative, highly therapeutic list, a distillation of some of the most critical and useful psychological concepts:

Truth #1: Emotions are not mysterious visitors; they can be identified and understood.

Truth #2: You can change your compulsive behaviors if you change your thoughts and address your feelings.

Truth #3:   Every behavior has an underlying purpose, and it's not always what we think.

Truth #4:   We all sabotage ourselves unless we confront our internal saboteur.

Truth #5:   All behavior requires permission so we must learn what we're permitting ourselves to do.

Truth #6:   Emotional energy is finite and needs to be invested, rather than wasted on wishing, worrying, and whining.

Truth #7:   Our relationships depend on self-empowerment and not on enabling others.

Truth #8:   Ego boundaries protect us from rejection, insult, and intimidation.

Truth #9:   You can trust people to be who they are, not who you want them to be.

Truth #10:   Time doesn't heal all pain; we heal ourselves by learning how to let go.

Some of these Truths may seem counterintuitive at first glance—for example, you may doubt that you sabotage yourself. Others may appear right on the mark, but you're unsure how to capitalize on them—for example, how do you create an ego boundary? Be assured that we'll help you understand their validity as well as how to apply them in your own life. For now, though, think of them as a type of psychological shorthand. If you ever wished for a manual that could help you understand your life, here it is. Too often, self-improvement efforts fall short because the methods used are overly complex and time-consuming or overly simplistic. These Truths offer a fast, comprehensible way to heal, solve problems, and find happiness.

For instance, take Truth #1. People often regret things they say in anger. They yell at their spouse or blow up at their boss, and they suffer the negative consequences. Yet these people sincerely believe that there isn't much they can do about these behaviors, because their feelings come on so quickly and so powerfully. "Feelings are facts," they say. Or they believe the psychological myth that you can't change how you feel. They may try to control their temper in these situations and have some sporadic success, but their feelings ultimately win out. They don't realize that if they investigate their anger and identify its origins and its triggers, they gain power over it.

In the next chapter, you'll learn how to do this.

Each chapter corresponds to a Truth, except the last one, which offers three different methods for you to apply all the Truths. In each chapter, you'll find explanations of that Truth, examples that illustrate these explanations, and exercises that allow you to practice using the Truth.

This is not a panacea, nor is it a substitute for therapy—you may have an issue that is deep-rooted and serious and requires professional help. Yet if you're like many of our patients, you want to contribute to your own learning and growth. You don't want to be a passive patient but an involved participant in the healing process. These Truths provide a way for you to become involved productively.

Thinking About Your Own Truths: Asking Some Essential Questions

Right from the start, we want you to start thinking in Truth terms. Ask yourself questions about how each Truth might apply to your own life. The goal isn't to answer the questions so much as to raise your psychological awareness. The more conscious you are of your thoughts and feelings, where they originate, the patterns they fall into, and how they impact your behaviors, the more able you will be to manage them effectively. This consciousness also helps prevent you from acting without thinking or becoming mired in feelings such as shame, anger, or sadness. Take a moment and think about the following set of questions, each of which is numbered and corresponds to a Truth:

1. Do you ever experience a feeling and aren't certain why you feel this way? Does it seem to come out of nowhere and impact not only your mood but your energy level, performance at work, and relationships with other people?

2. Are there certain ways in which you act compulsively? When you act this way, what are you usually thinking and what feelings are dominant?

3. Do you ever behave in a way that seems irrational or confusing? Do you say or do things that result in negative consequences, and, with hindsight, you can't believe what you said or did?

4. Have you acted in a way that hurt a relationship that you valued and wanted to keep strong? Have you ever done something in a work situation that ended up in your receiving a reprimand or led to your being fired? When you think about these situations, does it seem as if part of you wanted something bad to happen?

5. Are you aware of what you allow yourself to do? Have you ever examined what you deem as acceptable behavior from your family, friends, and work colleagues? Did you ever evaluate whether these behaviors should be permissible?

6. How much of a given day do you spend wishing, worrying, and whining? On a day when you've done a lot of wishing, worrying, and whining, do you feel exhausted? Does this feeling of emotional exhaustion prevent you from doing things that might be more productive?

7. Is there any one person whose actions have a major impact on your mood? Is there someone whose approval makes you feel great and/or whose disapproval makes you feel terrible? Do you sometimes feel at the mercy of what other people around you say and do?

8. Do you deal with criticism well? Can you separate who you are from how others act toward you? Are you able to handle rejection or insults without falling to pieces?

9. Do you sometimes try to change people and get them to act how you think they should act? Are you surprised when those closest to you behave in ways that run contrary to your expectations?

10. Do you depend on the passage of time to feel better after you've been emotionally hurt? Are you successful at letting go of a feeling that keeps you stuck or unproductive? Do you feel that you're able to work through emotional trauma and move on with your life?

In one sense, these are tough questions because they force you to confront challenging thoughts and feelings. They may make you anxious; they may cause you to consider events and issues that you'd rather not contemplate; and they may even cause you to go into denial. All of this is natural. In fact, it is necessary. You need to grapple with these things if you want to make progress. The good news is that we'll make grappling with them easier by giving you the information and coaching necessary to put the Truths behind the questions to good use.

Maximize the Value of What You're About to Learn

Personal growth does not occur merely by knowing about these Truths; your reflection and self-analysis are vital. Your willingness to complete the exercises in order to develop new skills will also be vital. By fostering new insights, developing more productive skills, and taking these Truths to heart, you will find your life to be more fulfilling. More than anything else, we hope you'll keep an open mind about what you're about to discover. We noted how the questions we asked can cause you to go into denial. They can also produce defensiveness and other forms of resistance. No one likes to admit that they've been sabotaging themselves or that they've been depending on someone else to make them happy, for instance. They can also prompt you to fall back on myths and misconceptions about yourself and the way your mind works.

If you make a concerted effort to get past your resistance to facing these psychological facts, however, you'll find that the effort is well worth it. These 10 Truths provide a map to a treasure trove of self-knowledge. They can help you find out why you always have problems with your boss, why you are overly dependent on alcohol to relieve your stress, and why your relationships—romantic and otherwise—haven't been what you hoped they would be. In other words, they can be used to address specific issues in your life and to formulate a plan for dealing with these issues more effectively. You will also gain a critical understanding of what drives you and what bedevils you, what stands in your way of achieving goals, and the strengths you have to help you realize them. The Truths can offer insights about who you are, why you are this way, and how you can become who you want to be. This is an ambitious objective, but the Truths are powerful tools. In the following pages, we'll give you the information, stories, and exercises that will help you use them effectively. (Note that all names and identifying details in this book have been changed to protect privacy.)

Chapter 1

Emotions Are Not Mysterious Visitors; They Can Be Identified and Understood

To different minds, the same world is Heaven and Hell.

—Anonymous

Happiness does not depend so much on circumstances as on one's inner self.

—Lady Randolph Churchill

Imagine if you could know your emotions as well as you know your thoughts. Consider what your life would be like if you could control your feelings rather than allowing them to control you. Instead of finding yourself ambushed by melancholy, you'd be able to connect this feeling to a specific trigger and source. Instead of blowing your top and yelling at a loved one or a boss, you'd be alert for when you were about to explode and could take steps to prevent it. You could prevent your feelings from sabotaging you, and you could experience positive emotions fully. Is this possible? Not only is it possible, but this Truth is achievable for just about anyone who puts in a bit of work. It doesn't require years of therapy. By understanding the sources, meanings, and physiology of your feelings, you can exert more power and control over them and lead a more fulfilling life.

Think about Jerry, who has a horrible temper. He flies off the handle at the slightest provocation, and this rage has destroyed his marriage, damaged his relationships with his children, and caused him to be fired from two jobs. At age 43, Jerry is resigned to his anger—he doesn't really understand why he becomes so furious and he wishes he could do something about his fury—but he figures, *That's just the way I am*. But Jerry doesn't have to be this way. If he makes an effort to figure out the source of his anger and the triggers that unleash it, he has an excellent chance of controlling it and preventing it from doing any more damage in his life. And, quite possibly, controlling this emotion could mean undoing at least some of the damage that has already been done.

Forget Jerry for the moment and consider an automobile. The manufacturer believes that our driving experience will be significantly enhanced if we know how the vehicle's features work, so the company provides a manual explaining these details. We might not read every word on every page—we probably have learned some of the details from owning other cars—but we're curious about the new, unfamiliar features and how they function. Perhaps it's our first car with anti-lock brakes—we learn we're not supposed to pump them to make them work effectively on a slick roadway, but that we should employ gentle pressure and they will engage. In the same way, we don't need a psychologist's understanding of emotions to control them. Learning about even one aspect of an emotion can be tremendously useful.

In his classic work, *The Road Less Traveled*, M. Scott Peck contends that emotions are slaves, and we are their masters. The odds are that this is not your experience or you wouldn't be reading this book. But you can be their master. It's not that complicated, and you don't need to be Freud to understand how emotions work. The first step is learning the five simple secrets about what emotions or feelings are all about:

s   All of our emotions are statements about us.

s   Our emotions are often the result of our thoughts, attitudes, and beliefs.

s   We are most emotional about the things in which we have the greatest investment.

s   Our emotions communicate how we perceive reality.

s   Emotions manifest themselves in three distinct forms.

Let's discuss these five pieces of psychological wisdom one at a time.

All of Our Emotions Are Statements About Us

Every emotion can be traced back to the way we process reality. As psychologists who treat clients who have experienced trauma and abuse, we often hear stories about the sexual abuse of children by adult caretakers. Though we've never experienced abuse personally, we undergo emotional and physiological changes when we listen to patients graphically detail the manner in which they were violated by trusted adults. We grit our teeth and clench our fists; we're powerfully angry. This anger is a statement about who we are. We perceive a terrible violation of power when adults use their positions of authority to abuse children, so our anger has to do with our thoughts and beliefs about abuse. Our anger emerges from who we are, both as individuals and as psychologists.

A retired physician, Dr. Charles, became a client when he was 85. A kind, compassionate gentleman with a quick, engaging smile, he told stories of more than 50 years of service as a general practitioner in rural America. Dr. Charles had a habit of describing people as "lovely." "He was a lovely fellow," "she was a lovely woman." Consider why he used this word. The reason he found everyone to be so lovely was that he himself was so loving. Dr. Charles's warm and compassionate feelings toward so many people were statements about him.

Now consider how you feel when you're driving. You may be hypercautious and inclined to obey every traffic signal and sign, yielding the right of way to other vehicles to avoid potential danger. Or perhaps you're at the other end of the emotional spectrum, navigating the roads as if they were a racetrack and speeding constantly. Or maybe you're one of those people who drive with a sense of entitlement, feeling angry when people cut you off or when someone in front of you is driving too slowly for your liking. Just think about your feelings at a yellow light: If you're driver A, you feel caution; if you're driver B, you feel challenge and excitement; and if you're driver C, you feel frustration and anger. Thus, the light literally signals your emotions. You can use these signals to help figure out how your mindset creates your emotions.

Our Emotions Are Often the Results of Our Thoughts, Attitudes, and Beliefs

A man lies fast asleep on a city sidewalk, half-in, half-out of a cardboard box. His face rests on the arm of his flannel shirt; drool falls on his sleeve. Four pedestrians walk by. The first one notices the sleeping man's pitiful condition but looks away. *I didn't see anything*, he thinks, as he continues his morning walk without another thought of the man on the sidewalk. The second pedestrian spots the man in his peripheral vision and says to himself, *There but for the grace of God go I. That man could have been me in my days of out-of-control partying. I have much to be grateful for*. Then he makes a beeline for work and offers a silent prayer for the unfortunate man in the cardboard box. The third pedestrian has a far different response to the sleeping man. He goes on an inner tirade: *It's lazy, good-for-nothing bums like him that lie around and sleep on the street who are bringing down this country. Here I am working my butt off to make an honest living, and my tax dollars are being used to support people like him. Doesn't he have any pride?* The fourth passerby looks in horror when he first sees the sleeping man. *Oh, that poor soul*, he thinks, as he walks to the side of the homeless gent. He checks to see if the man is alive, wondering if the elements had overcome him and what he can do to help. He finally decides to let the man sleep as he gently places a 20-dollar bill in his shirt pocket. He prays for the man throughout the day. The sleeping man becomes a profoundly sad image permanently etched in his memory, an ever-present reminder of the plight of the less fortunate.

Each passerby projects his particular thoughts, attitudes, and beliefs onto the sleeping man. They are very different people, and so each one interprets the stimulus of the sleeping man through his own worldview. Their perceptions are their reality, and so it is for all of us. Perceptions, thoughts, attitudes, and beliefs are more important in the creation of emotion than the reality itself. Therefore, don't make the mistake of believing that your emotions emerge from particular situations, experiences, or people. As William Shakespeare wrote, "Things are neither good nor bad, but thinking makes it so." Thousands of years earlier, King Solomon mused in the Book of Proverbs, "How a man thinketh in his heart, so is he." Later, the philosopher Epictetus wrote, "Men are disturbed not by things, but by the principles and notions which they form concerning things."

Consider this story from *The Big Little Book of Jewish Wit and Wisdom* (Black Dog & Leventhal, 2000). Sadie's husband, Jake, had been slipping in and out of a coma for several months, yet his faithful wife stayed by his bedside day and night. One night Jake awoke and motioned for her to come closer. He said, "My Sadie, you have been with me through all the bad times. When I got fired, you were there to support me. When my business failed, you were there. When I got shot, you were by my side. When we lost the house, you gave me support. When my health failed, you were still by my side. You know what, Sadie?" "What, dear?" she asked gently. "I think you are bad luck." Jake's perceptions of reality, not the facts or circumstances, created his emotions.

Perception, much more than the base reality of events, governs our emotions. For instance, if we think our lover is cheating on us, that perception is what causes us to be angry, sad, and so on. It doesn't matter that he's not cheating and that we just made an erroneous assumption. Similarly, if he is cheating but we don't know it, we may be happy as a clam. Again, it's perception that impacts our emotional state.

On Ash Wednesday 2004, New Market Films released the controversial movie, *The Passion of the Christ*. The film depicted the director's interpretation of the final 12 hours of the life of Jesus Christ. One reporter, Abby Weingarten, highlighted the intense and varied responses of moviegoers in an article in which she interviewed people of different faiths and philosophies *(Herald-Tribune*, March 4, 2004*)*. A Protestant minister remarked on how the movie accurately portrayed Christ's love for all mankind. A rabbi believed the movie was anti-Semitic. It reminded her of her childhood when young schoolmates threw rocks at her and yelled, "Dirty Jew, you killed Jesus!" A Muslim spokesperson claimed he and other Muslims would not see the film because showing the torture and death of the prophet Jesus was disrespectful. A reverend of the Unitarian Universalist Church felt the movie depicted graphic violence for "commercial reasons."

I worked with a woman who at age 76 was permanently blinded by a physician during a routine medical procedure. This woman was understandably sad and frustrated at her inability to carry out the normal activities of daily living that she had been accustomed to doing. Nonetheless, she didn't wallow in self-pity. Instead, humility and gratitude were her defining traits. She was a source of inspiration to her friends and family. The fact that she believed she had been blessed with love, support, and prayers instead of seeing herself as a helpless victim was a statement about her and the way that she processed reality. No doubt, others in a similar situation would be bitter and resentful. Yet this woman embraced positive emotions. Indeed, researchers have discovered that happy people tend to remain happy even after sustaining great losses such as blindness or paralysis. They emerge as happy blind or paralyzed people. Similarly, unhappy people who win the lottery and become wealthy are often still unhappy.

University of Pennsylvania psychologist Dr. Martin Seligman conducted research that suggests that people explain reality to themselves in a predictable fashion (he calls it an *explanatory style*). According to his research, a self-deprecatory or demoting mindset is a major player in clinical depression. Consider the case of a man I met several years ago who had been diagnosed with a *dysthymic disorder* (chronic, low-grade depression). Alan had been treated with medication ever since he returned from a tour of duty in Vietnam. When I asked him about the beginnings of his depression, Alan could pinpoint the exact date and time when he crashed—the fall of Saigon in 1975. As he watched the North Vietnamese takeover of the city on his living room television set, he drew two immediate conclusions: 1) all of his efforts in Vietnam had been in vain, and 2) he was a complete failure. His perception was that he was a loser who would always underachieve. Alan was not able to see that he had not failed in Vietnam; his negative perception was more powerful than his reality. As long as he believed he was a failure, he would remain an unhappy and unproductive man.

Like many of us, Alan viewed himself as a victim. You don't have to participate in a losing war to develop this attitude. You can lose a job or get divorced and adopt this same negative perception. What's worth understanding, though, is that negative "victim emotions" (such as Alan's depression) come from us, not from external events. It may seem like a small thing, but when we realize that we have control over how we feel, we react to events differently. Yes, it's sad that we lost our job, but we don't have to let our former employer's bad year or a boss we didn't get along with turn us into a worthless mope. How we think about what happens to us—our attitudes and beliefs about a given event—is what governs our emotional reaction.

Alan recognized this Truth in therapy, and he made a concerted effort to change his perceptions. He came to the conclusion that he was not a failure or a loser. He stopped taking responsibility for the outcome of the war and began to rethink his attitude of self-loathing. As a result, he was able to climb out of the depressive pit he had occupied for more than a decade!

We Are Most Emotional About the Things in Which We Have the Greatest Investment

Feelings can describe who we are: happy-go-lucky child, angry old man, anxious woman. They also speak to our investments—where we put our emotional energy. Have you ever watched a TV awards ceremony in which the announcer excitedly described an actress's dress on the red carpet, and you wondered how anyone could care that much about someone else's clothing? Or thought about why 50,000 people would pack a stadium and cheer like crazy for a football team with a 2-9 record? Or cried at every sappy movie? Or been devoted to a job that requires 70 hours of work a week and doesn't pay all that well? Or been married to someone who seems rude and mean-spirited? People are invested in many different facets of life—family, money, sports, sex, cars, clothes, and so on—all of which have the power to contribute to their emotions. In fact, all of our emotions are statements about our investments. If we feel something, we are invested. If we feel strongly, we are very invested.

What do you think about the upcoming election for mayor in Albuquerque? Unless you happen to live there, you probably don't care.

You'll have no emotional reaction to the election. Why? Because without investment, there will be no emotion. If you don't invest, you won't feel. Stop a moment and consider the things that make you feel most intensely. What things matter most to you? Is it your job, your looks, your spouse, your children, your wealth, your status, your success, your hobbies? The correlation between investment and emotion provides you with insight into what really matters, both for yourself and for others. It's not always what people say that matters most. Sometimes, people insist that their job is the most important thing in their life, yet when they talk about it, they are very matter-of-fact; they never rhapsodize about a new project or talk passionately about a goal they've achieved. In fact, they reserve their most emotional statements for their weekend hobby. That's a pretty clear clue that they've been fooling themselves and others about what really matters to them.

Using emotion as a barometer of what's important can help you make important life decisions. For instance, you're dating a guy who claims what matters most to him is family; he says that he wants to have children, that he relishes time he spends with his nephews, and that he's close to his parents and siblings. Yet in the six months you've been going with him, he rarely tells you a story about family in which he manifests any strong emotion. He never tears up when talking about a beloved cousin who died young; and when he has a disagreement with his father about a business matter, he doesn't become angry or upset in any way (negative emotions are also signs of what matters). On the other hand, he becomes tremendously worked up—expressing both positive and negative emotions—when talking about financial strategies that paid off as well as ones that didn't. Thus, these emotional reactions give you insight into his value system.

Other factors play a role in how people express emotions. Some people are more low-key emotionally than others, and it's difficult to discern any strong feelings about anything. In fact, many people have trouble reading what's important to them. For instance, John is convinced he should go to law school. His father and mother are lawyers, he scored well on the law school standardized tests, and he has always thought about the benefits of becoming a lawyer—the prestige, the money, and so on. Yet when John considers how he feels about being a lawyer, he realizes that there's very little emotion. In fact, he exhibits strong feelings when thinking and talking about other areas of his life—white water rafting, hiking, and travel. He is heavily invested in all these so-called recreational activities, but he only has an intellectual investment in being a lawyer. The investment-emotion correlation provides a measure for something that is not always easy to read otherwise.

Our Emotions Communicate How We Perceive Reality

Our emotions are innate messengers that provide information to us about how we perceive reality. Unfortunately, we may misinterpret these messages or feel too emotional to appreciate what they are telling us. What does it mean when we feel terribly sad or when we become furious? Here are some interpretations of common emotional responses:

Anxiety

Anxiety, the nervous feeling we have that may include racing heart, unsettled stomach, constriction of the chest, dry mouth, and hand tremors—is something most of us experience at one time or another. Sometimes we can identify its source—an upcoming performance review at work, for instance—and sometimes it's a vague and unidentifiable feeling. Even when we knew the source of our anxiety, however, the emotional message is incomplete. If we want to gain a full understanding of our anxiety, we need to look at it as a perceived threat to our investment.

The formula is Investment + Threat = Anxiety. For example, if you have relatives who died from colon cancer and you're going to have your first colonoscopy, you have an investment (you value your life) and a threat (the test may reveal something that could kill you). On other hand, if you're going to the doctor and he takes your blood pressure, and you have no history of high blood pressure, then you'll feel little, if any, anxiety. In some instances, you may see a threat but not feel anxious because you lack an investment. Of course, if you're dealing with medical tests, you're invested because you value your life. Threats in other areas, however, can be inconsequential based on your particular perspective. A downturn in real estate value does not typically induce anxiety in people who do not own property. Consider this adage: "It's a recession when your neighbor is unemployed; it's a depression when you're unemployed." The degree of relevance to you determines your perception of reality and, hence, your emotional response.

Anxiety, then, is not necessarily a clinical problem as much as it is a message to the self *from* the self that something we value is being threatened. Examining our anxiety from an investment/threat framework is helpful, in that it gives us the information we need to deal with the source of our anxiety. Without this framework, however, we respond counterproductively to our anxiety. For instance, we may medicate anxiety by drinking alcohol or taking a tranquilizer. It is akin to driving a car, seeing the oil light come on indicating we're a quart or more low, and asking our passenger to remove a hammer from the glove compartment and smashing the light. We're eliminating the anxiety-producing message without dealing with the underlying problem. As a result, your car will break down if you keep on driving; and you may suffer some sort of breakdown if you don't address the source of your anxiety.

Use your anxiety to understand how you're perceiving reality. Figure out your investment and the threat to that investment. In this way, you can face the source of what is making you so fearful and nervous. Research from the University of Texas (Powers, 1994) concludes that the best way to overcome anxiety is to face the source of it directly. Ignoring or escaping the anxiety tends to result in more anxiety in the future, and it prolongs it as well. Therefore, if you're anxious about flying in airplanes, face into it by gritting your teeth and flying. If you're anxious about speaking in public, give a speech. You don't have to take a flight around the world or schedule a speech in front of 1,000 people. Start off small—take a short flight, or talk to a small group on a subject you know well.

Sadness

With sadness, the message is different. We perceive the loss of something valuable. The death of a loved one, the end of a job or the breakup of a relationship can create sadness. Sadness is not the same as clinical depression, which is marked by at least two weeks of symptoms such as the "blues," insomnia, feelings of hopelessness and/or worthlessness, apathy, the loss of pleasure in what were once rewarding activities, decrease in libido, and a decrease or increase in appetite. Although sadness can be a part of clinical depression, it is a normal human emotion. As long as you can function and the sadness diminishes and disappears through time, you're not depressed. The key here is to identify the valuable thing that has been lost. Sometimes, we're afraid to admit why we're feeling sad—we don't want to admit that our ex's departure hurt us, for example—and sometimes, we tend to assign superficial reasons for our sadness—it's a cold, gray day—rather than focus on what has been lost.

Guilt

We do not feel guilty when we do something wrong. We feel guilty when we think we have done something wrong. The message: We perceive that we've violated our moral code. Consider the following example. Two men are fishing on a beautiful Sunday morning on a calm sea. One man is enjoying the placid waters and azure skies while the other is plagued with an irritating sense of guilt; he perceives he has violated his moral code. The guilty man was born and raised in a family that emphasized that one needs to be in church on Sunday morning. Hence, it is the perception of wrongdoing, not the actual behavior, that creates the emotion of guilt.

Guilt helps us examine the validity of our moral code. This man, for instance, is denying himself the pleasure of a Sunday morning in a beautiful environment. If he examines his moral code and finds it valid, he should change his behavior and spend Sundays in church. If, however, he finds that his morality is an artifice created by a puritanical upbringing, then he should adjust his moral code and allow himself this pleasure.

In order to feel guilty, and in order to develop the capacity to make choices according to a moral standard, we must first learn the difference between right and wrong. When we violate this knowledge and standard, we experience feelings of guilt. There are people who are guilt sponges. They feel guilty about everything around them as if they had control over the weather, the economy, and the traffic. Others feel no guilt despite stealing huge amounts of money from a corporation or even committing murder. Again, it is not the behavior, but the belief and belief system that fosters feelings of guilt.

Those who feel guilty about everything were often taught at a young age that they were responsible for particular events as well as the feelings and behaviors of others. They may have received blame for external events over which they had no control, and therefore learned to be overly vigilant. Hence, their journey through life is fraught with the irrational belief that they must worry about everything. On the opposite end of the spectrum lies the sociopath—someone who violates the law without regard for others. All of life is perceived as an extension of him- or herself. The sociopath has no remorse, guilt, or empathy for others.

Panic

People compare panic attacks to the sensation of dying and/or having a heart attack. They note symptoms such as powerful constriction in the chest, racing heart, rapid and shallow breathing, tingling sensations in the arms and legs, hypersensitivity to light and sound, weak knees, gastrointestinal disturbance, and a powerful need to get out or escape from some place or experience. Panic attacks (also called anxiety attacks) are far more intense than the generalized feeling of anxiety described earlier and are a very common problem in our society, affecting a significant percentage of the population. Panic disorder is defined by having two or three of these attacks within a month and/or being preoccupied with thoughts of having them. Although some people require tranquilizers or antidepressants to deal with panic attacks, we've found that this powerful emotional reaction can be controlled when people understand the message of these attacks: feeling trapped and/or out of control. In fact, it is the core message. Invariably, our clients report this perception as preceding an attack.

For instance, a physician who had never experienced a panic attack in his life was scuba diving. This was an enjoyable adventure until he went inside a cave to explore the underwater sea life. It wasn't what he found in the cave as much as what he didn't (the exit) that precipitated his very first panic attack. Another gentleman in his 60s had his first panic attack during a cardiac procedure in which a heavy machine was placed on his chest—a little too close for his comfort. When he found there was no one in the room and he believed he couldn't move the machine, he experienced his first panic attack.

Feeling trapped is not based solely on our physical circumstances, however. Another retired man was hospitalized for persistent panic attacks—something he had never experienced in his life until retirement. He had sold his house in Chicago and bought one in Florida, much to the delight of his wife. He, on the other hand, found that he hated living in Florida. He could see no way out; he felt trapped, which resulted in the attacks. It's pertinent to note that panic attacks frequently occur in grocery stores when people are in line waiting to pay, or in crowded movie theaters where all the seats around the person are occupied. Restaurants with no easy exits, airplanes, and traffic jams all pose a potential threat to someone who suffers from panic disorder.

Understanding this dynamic can help people deal effectively with their panic attacks. Instead of thinking of them as coming out of nowhere or as a result of excessive stress, we need to grasp what makes us feel trapped and recognize that this is a perception rather than a reality, and that the condition is only temporary, and that it poses no serious risk. This is a much better way of dealing with this type of emotional chaos than avoidance. Avoiding situations that trigger panic attacks may offer temporary relief, but this escapist behavior provides no long-term resolution for the attacks. Invariably, the panic attacks return because the core emotional message has been ignored.

Anger

Anger seems simple enough on the surface. We know the people in our lives who make us angriest (our kids, our spouse, our parents, our boss), and we know what it is they do they makes us angry (they defy us, they order us around, and so on). But what we don't know, and what is essential to understand, is what this emotion is telling us. Anger often emerges from a perception of having been violated. For example, when we are cut off in traffic, we may feel anger toward the other driver. Similarly, if someone flirts with our spouse, reads our diary without permission, or shares our personal secrets, we may also feel angry.

A variation on this theme is when our expectations are violated—we expect a positive result, and instead we get a negative one. Experiencing rain six out of seven days on a vacation makes some people angry, given their expectations of sun and fun. Expecting a thank-you note after a wedding gift, flowers on an anniversary, or a promotion or raise after a year of service may lead to anger when these expectations aren't met.

It's normal to become angry on occasion, but anger becomes a counterproductive emotion when its frequency, intensity, or duration is beyond the norm. You have constant temper tantrums (frequency); you are verbally or physically abusive (intensity); you are furious for hours instead of minutes (duration), making it difficult to maintain a relationship. Typically, people who are overly angry make excuses—they blame their anger on other people, events, and situations. What they fail to understand is that the cause of their anger is internal, not external. It is their perception of these externals that causes their anger. When they perceive that a violation has occurred—a friend didn't play fair in a game of tennis, a business partner didn't deliver a project by the date he promised—they are enraged.

Trying to manage anger by moderating behavior when we reach the boiling point is an ineffective way to handle this powerful emotion. It's much more effective to understand the perception of violation to which you're vulnerable and to learn to think differently about it, thus preventing the anger from reaching that point in the first place.

Other emotions exist besides these five, but the goal is always to grasp how a given emotion arises based on a perception of reality. For instance:

s   Envy emerges when we perceive we're inferior to someone and are unable to accept the perceived inferiority.

s   Shame hits us when we perceive ourselves to be bad or worthless.

s   Pride fills us when we perceive that we've accomplished something significant.

It may seem like a simple thing, but recognizing that emotions begin with perceptions is easy to forget in the heat of daily battles. When we don't remember the role perception plays, we often act in ways that hurt ourselves or others.

Emotions Manifest Themselves in Three Distinct Forms

An emotion is a three-headed creature. If we are to fully understand what we're feeling, we need to consider its three aspects:

1. The subjective experience (feelings).
2. The physiological expression (biological changes).
3. The behavioral communication (our words and deeds).

First, how we feel is our subjective, individualized, and personal experience of the world. We use words as reference points by which we label our mental and physical reactions to events based upon our history. For example, you and your spouse may see a movie together, and you may describe it as sappy, whereas your spouse may call it heartfelt. You cannot expect others to feel the same way you do, even if the other person is your spouse. You may share some common feelings, but your relationships will be much better if you accept that feelings are subjective and they're articulated in different ways. In this way, you won't be resentful when someone doesn't feel the same way as you do. As the saying goes, variety is the spice of life. Different perspectives make life interesting. They are normal, and not a matter of right and wrong.

Second, our emotions can be explained physiologically. The word emotion comes from the Latin word *emovere*, which means stir up, agitate, excite, or move. Emotions are more than a state of mind. They involve a series of complex physical reactions, including hormonal release, increased blood flow, and neurons firing in the brain. These physical changes occur within two branches of the central nervous system (CNS). The sympathetic branch of the CNS mobilizes the body into action; nervous impulses travel from the brain and spinal cord to various organs. The parasympathetic branch of the CNS conserves energy and resources. The sympathetic branch is employed during the "flight or fight" reaction when situations are perceived as stressful. This internal activity leads to changes such as the dilation of pupils, perspiration, increased heart rate, and dry mouth. The adrenal glands, located just above the kidneys, secrete the hormone adrenaline, which causes dilation of air passages to the lungs (think rapid, shallow breathing), increased heart rate (pounding in your chest), increased blood pressure, and a slowing of the digestive process.

Think of it as the body's self-contained emergency system. When we perceive something as very scary, such as hearing footsteps behind us on a dark abandoned street, our body prepares us to make a run for it. If those footsteps result in an unavoidable confrontation, those same internal changes would prepare us for battle. Notice that the blood flow increases to the major muscle groups (arms, legs, back, chest) preparing us to fight or flee. The blood flow decreases to other parts of the anatomy—the digestive and reproductive systems, for example—presumably because they are considerably less important when survival is on the line. Hence, during times of prolonged stress, food is left undigested, and sexual activity/performance is compromised. When men just think about stressful situations, the flow of blood is directed away from the penis and toward the major muscle groups. When the perceived threat subsides and the flight or fight response is no longer necessary, the parasympathetic branch of the CNS returns the body to normal, a state known as *homeostasis*. Equilibrium or balance is restored in the body, with breathing rate, heart rate, and blood pressure all returning to normal.

In the brain, the flight or fight reaction is processed in the limbic system, especially in the area known as the *amygdala*. Less intense emotions, especially those not resulting from a perceived threat, are processed in the pre-frontal cortex of the brain. Interestingly, damage to either area (pre-frontal cortex or amygdala) will cause us to lose our ability to understand, express, and control our emotions.

Why is all of this important? Because you may not recognize how much your emotions impact your physical state—and vice versa. As a result, guys may become terribly depressed when high stress results in impotence, and women may become upset when stress causes them digestive difficulties. Poor management of anger has been associated with the onset of heart disease and some cancers. Grief and unresolved sadness may lead to system immunosuppression, resulting in a reduced capacity to fend off illness, decline in work productivity, depression, and suicide. People often give lip service to the mind-body connection, but they don't always recognize the relationship in their own lives. Use your body as a sophisticated, sensitive warning system. If you're feeling sluggish, if some body part isn't working properly, or if you have headaches, consider the possibility that your body is trying to tell you something about your emotional state.

Third, expect your emotions to drive certain behaviors. When we laugh, yell, cry, smile, make sarcastic remarks, or become aggressive, this behavior is a consequence of emotion. Behavior is a tremendously useful expression of how we're feeling. It is a brilliant communication tool, a way to release the emotion inside of us and relieve the pressure of that emotion. If we're "bursting" with happiness, we need to laugh, shout thanks to the heavens, and do a little dance. If we're filled with sorrow, we need to cry. Not only does this release help us, it lets others know how we're feeling. In this way, we receive their kind words and gestures, or they share with us in our celebrations.

If you try to separate your emotions from your behaviors—if you don't act the way you feel—you're probably not going to be a particularly happy or fulfilled person. All of us need to express our feelings in behaviors. It's not enough just to say we're happy or we're sad. In fact, to understand and experience our emotions fully, we need to combine the subjective, the physiological, and the behavioral. If we can appreciate the subjective nature of feelings, recognize their physical aspect, and express them through behavior, we'll function much more effectively in the world—and feel a lot better about ourselves. We'll get more into how to control these behaviors in the next Chapter.

Exercises

This first Truth is all about getting to know your emotions. We've tried to take the mystery out of common emotions such as fear, anger, and sadness, and we hope you now have a much better understanding of why you feel the way you do and what these feelings mean. To help you apply this learning to your own life, we've created four exercises, starting with one that may surprise you with the range of feelings you experience.

Exercise 1—How Did You Feel?

This exercise is designed to get you in touch with your full emotional spectrum. You may not realize how wide-ranging your emotions are, so the questions here will make you aware of this. As you'll see, the questions refer to events that occurred in your past. If a given question is not relevant—for example, if you never experienced the death of a pet—change the question so that it's speculative: How would you feel *if* your pet died?

1. How did you feel when your best friend moved away?

    _____

2. How did you feel when you earned your highest test score?

    _____

3. How did you feel when your dog/cat passed away?

    _____

4. How did you feel when your parents fought?

    _____

5. How did you feel when you were falsely accused of something you didn't do?

    _____

6. How did you feel when a friend shared a secret of yours?

    _____

7. How did you feel when other students wouldn't let you join them?

    _____

8. How did you feel when you were promoted?

    _____

9. How did you feel when your father was drunk and your friends were visiting?

    _____

10. How did you feel when you vacationed at your favorite place?

    _____

11. How did you feel when someone threatened to harm you?

    _____

12. How did you feel when someone you know told a lie about you?

    _____

13. How did you feel when your family and friends visited you in the hospital?

    _____

14. How did you feel when your parents broke a promise to you?

    _____

15. How did you feel when your parents compared you to other children?

    _____

16. How did you feel when no one picked you to be on their team?

    _____

17. How did you feel when all your hard work paid off?

    _____

18. How did you feel when you were selected for a job you wanted?

    _____

19. How did you feel when you thought of your mother?

_____

20. How did you feel when a loved one let you down?

_____

21. How did you feel when you couldn't stop thinking bad thoughts?

_____

22. How did you feel when you finished the race?

_____

Exercise 2—What Causes You to Feel That Way?

Understanding your feelings means digging below the surface to identify the cause of those feelings. Here, we'd like you to fill in the blanks with a specific event, situation, or relationship that produces the listed feeling:

1. I feel excited when _____

_____

2. I feel sad when _____

_____

3. I feel embarrassed when _____

_____

4. I feel nervous when _____

_____

5. I feel jealous when _____

_____

6. I feel happy whenever _____

_____

7. I feel depressed after _____

_____

8. I feel apprehensive when _____

_____

9. I feel upset every time _____

_____

10. I feel confused when _____

_____

11. I feel loved when _____

_____

12. I lose interest when _____

_____

13. I feel proud whenever _____

_____

14. I feel irritable because_____

_____

15. I become incensed whenever _____

_____

Exercise 3—Getting to the Bottom of Anger

Anger is always a secondary emotion. It is the result of something happening that you wish had not happened or something that did not happen that you wish had occurred. Here, identify the cause of your anger, rather than dwelling in that negative emotion. Fill in the blanks with a situation that's recent and relevant, and describe why you feel the way you do:

I am so angry because _____

_____

I resent him/her because _____

_____

It ticks me off that _____

_____

I get so frustrated when _____

_____

I can't believe that you _____

_____

I have been so upset ever since you_____

_____

Exercise 4—Your Top Five Investments

Fill in your top five emotional investments in the space below, and write down the biggest threat to that investment you could imagine. For instance, your major investment could be in your spouse, and the biggest threat to that investment could be the possibility of divorce. Doing this exercise will help you become clear on what really matters to you emotionally, and what "unknowns" make you the most anxious.

	INVESTMENT	THREAT
1.		
2.		
3.		
4.		
5.		

Chapter 2

You Can Change
Your Compulsive Behaviors
If You Change Your Thoughts and
Address Your Feelings

It's choice—not chance—that determines your destiny.

—Jean Nidetch,
founder of Weight Watchers International

Lord, help me to be the kind of person my psychiatrist medicates me to be.

—Laurie Rosin, editor

Now that you have become aware of our previous Truth that emotions can be understood and even controlled to some extent, you may wonder whether it's really possible to change the behaviors these emotions produce. Think about what you do when you feel terribly sad or incredibly angry. If you're deeply sad, you may sit and watch numerous stupid television shows. When you are incredibly angry, you may verbally or physically abuse people you care about—or you may adopt behaviors that are self-destructive. You know these behaviors are counterproductive. You may even want to stop them. And yet, your emotions are so powerful that they hold you in a viselike grip, creating behavioral responses that are utterly predictable—and utterly compulsive.

Many of us have compulsions. We drink too much when we're sad; we chain-smoke when we're anxious; we have temper tantrums when we're angry; we cheat on our spouses when we're feeling lonely. These compulsive behaviors can take many forms, but they're always triggered by an intense emotional state. Sarah, 45, was abandoned by her parents as a child. Additionally, a male relative sexually abused her when she was seven years old. As a result of these experiences, Sarah has always felt ashamed, frightened, and vulnerable to being hurt by men. To deal with these intense feelings, Sarah chose a compulsive behavior as a form of self-medication. Specifically, Sarah became a compulsive eater. If she felt rejected by her husband or her child defied her, she sought comfort in a package of cookies. If her male boss criticized her work performance, she got together with her favorite companions, Ben and Jerry. Comfort foods consoled Sara when she felt worthless, ineffectual, or unloved.

We'll return to Sarah's story a bit later. For now, recognize that it is possible to escape the cycle of compulsive behavior. It's fortunate that obsessions and anxiety are not terminal conditions. They may flood your mind with troubling thoughts, but they don't have to control your behaviors. In fact, when you grasp what emotion is producing these behaviors, and the underlying dynamic of how and why it is causing you to act in a specific way, you can learn to control them.

Compulsive Behaviors: Short-Term Relief for Long-Term Pain

When you act compulsively, you engage in activities that change your emotional state—seemingly for the better, but they actually produce significant problems in the long run. When you watch TV or play video games compulsively, for example, you may relieve the immediate anxiety you're suffering from; you escape into virtual worlds and the problems of TV show characters. In the long term, however, this compulsive behavior may prevent you from dealing with the real source of your anxiety. In some people there exists a driving force so powerful that it causes them to engage in behaviors that have serious negative consequences. Sarah was psychologically, and possibly physically, addicted to food. She gave herself an emotional fix, a temporary release from the pain that relationships caused her. We need to understand how these compulsions function because that will help us learn to change the emotion that throws us into our particular compulsive activities. Therefore, consider that compulsive behaviors:

▶ Alter feelings.

▶ Work as a temporary remedy.

▶ Persist despite negative consequences.

▶ Take on a life of their own.

▶ Follow a predictable pattern.

Compulsive behaviors alter feelings

Compulsive behaviors help us feel something we want to feel and/or stop us from feeling what we do not want to feel. People who step out of a tense meeting at work to smoke a cigarette do so in an effort to relieve tension and to replace the tension with a more relaxed feeling. Happy hours across the country are attended by people who have a need to put aside some of the pressures and frustrations of the work week. They also yearn to feel something—the alcohol-induced "buzz"—that they would not feel if they drove directly home. Workaholics report a great sense of accomplishment at conquering projects. Older men who engage in affairs with younger women feel desirable and rejuvenated.

Each person is compulsive in a way suited to his or her particular needs, lifestyle, and genetic makeup. For instance, one of my high-achieving patients told me he uses cocaine to burn the candle at both ends. Sarah chose food in part to feel less attractive to men as she gained weight. The less attractive she believed she was, the safer she would be from the unwanted advances of abusive males. The adult child of parents who were neurotic about trying to keep him safe from harm may grow up to be a compulsive risk-taker, gambling in relationships, business, and in Las Vegas.

Compulsive behaviors work as a temporary remedy

I have yet to talk to a patient who compulsively smokes banana peels. Perhaps some people have attempted this in an act of desperation or novelty, but I can't imagine anyone doing it obsessively. Smoking banana peels is not an issue for people because it doesn't work. We do not get high from smoking banana peels, nor do they help us forget our problems. Crack cocaine, on the other hand, is highly effective in providing a high and a temporary escape from reality. When it comes to the reduction of anxiety, alcohol is also very effective (though, of course, drug and alcohol abuse create all sorts of other problems). When a behavior meets a need, it is likely to continue. People repeat behaviors that work.

Mood-altering substances known as *endorphins* stimulate the pleasure centers of the brain. A flood of these brain chemicals is released, which creates euphoric sensations. Joggers claim that endorphins are released during their runs, resulting in what is known as a runner's high. These chemical reactions in the brain provide a brief state of pleasure, and escape from the perceived stress. A wide variety of behaviors provide a temporary balm for emotional pain. For some people, shopping offers relief—not an occasional trip to the store, but long, frequent, compulsive trips in search of specific items, or just to buy anything at all. The shopping routine is calming. It distracts them from the emotional hurt they suffered and allows them to concentrate on something else. With every purchase comes a sense of accomplishment, of being in control. Other compulsive behaviors may involve surfing the net, playing video games, or devoting one's free time to celebrity watching. All of it works, but it only works for a while and at a great long-term cost.

Compulsive behaviors persist despite negative consequences

Sarah was well aware that she was more than 100 pounds overweight. In response to her physician's gentle prodding, she said, "I know, I know. I need to lose weight." Cigarette smokers have been aware of the dangers of their addiction for more than four decades now. Compulsive gamblers persist in their attempts to score the big one, in spite of a painful history of bankruptcies, foreclosures, and broken relationships. People shop compulsively and run up huge credit card charges that they have no hope of ever paying. Others waste enormous amounts of time watching television shows to avoid having to do homework, search for a job, exercise, or anything productive.

Why do people engage in these behaviors despite the negative consequences? This question has plagued researchers and clinicians for years. Contrary to what you might think, it's not because they're weak or lack willpower. Most people are aware that shopping 20 hours a week is not good for them, and they'll sometimes try to reduce or stop the behavior. Yet, despite their intense efforts, they often fail. That's because they've developed a physiological or psychological dependence on the behavior, and this dependence segues into something else—something that intensifies its hold.

Compulsive behaviors take on a life of their own

Gordon Allport, an internationally known psychologist, coined the term *functional autonomy*. This term describes how certain behaviors begin for one reason but then develop the autonomy necessary to continue on their own, long after the original reason is no longer present. For example, a young girl starts smoking cigarettes at age 13 to fit in with a group of peers. At age 46, this woman is still smoking cigarettes even though the original reason is no longer a factor. (Ironically, she may receive even more pressure from her middle-aged peers to quit smoking than she did from her teen peer group to start.) She persists in smoking because the behavior has taken on a life of its own. Biochemically addicted to the nicotine and psychologically reliant on its stress-reducing capability, she relishes the feeling of well-being she receives from smoking, and the feeling she gets from rewarding herself with a cigarette after not having had one for a few hours. Even though she no longer needs to smoke in order to be cool or fit in with a certain group of people, she sees herself as a smoker. If she were to create a dictionary definition for herself, smoker, would be one of the adjectives she would use.

In fact, people also define themselves as shoppers, as Brad Pitt fans, as video game players, as workout kings or queens. Initially, these behaviors help mitigate an uncomfortable or painful feeling, but over time, they cease to serve that function. Instead, they have their own *gestalt*, a particular set of qualities that contribute to how into how an individual sees him- or herself. When compulsions become the behavior by which you define yourself, they are difficult to give up.

Compulsive behaviors follow a predictable pattern

If you want to break the hold your compulsions have on you, you'll need to recognize their patterns. Dr. Paul McHugh, director of psychiatry at the Johns Hopkins University, theorized that compulsive behaviors fall into the category of motivated behaviors, cyclical in nature and predictable in their form. The cycle of motivated behaviors is a four-part process, and understanding how you move through this process diminishes their power. Once you plug your specific behaviors into the following four-step pattern, you can identify how they evolved and where you can intervene to get them under control. You'll become aware of why you engage in these behaviors and how they offer only temporary rewards. You'll see how you became caught in the cycle:

Now let's see how Sarah's compulsive eating fits into these four stages.

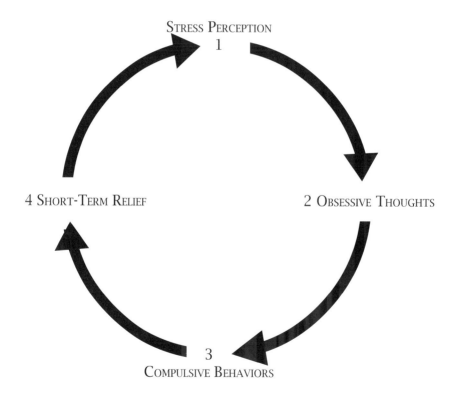

STRESS PERCEPTION
1

2 OBSESSIVE THOUGHTS

3
COMPULSIVE BEHAVIORS

4 SHORT-TERM RELIEF

Stage 1—Stress Perception: At Stage 1, Sarah perceives some external event in her life as unacceptable, unmanageable, or emotionally undesirable. This may be her husband's cold, detached, unappreciative tendencies or her child's disrespectful and defiant behaviors.

Stage 2—Obsessive Thoughts: Here Sarah initiates an internal dialogue with herself, often without being aware of it. Her thoughts and self-statements revolve around her loss of control, resulting in further belittling thoughts. Without long-term coping skills to manage either the perceived stress or her negative thoughts, she is compelled to act. Her options for action are short-term avoidance strategies—more specifically, overeating.

Stage 3—Compulsive Behaviors: Sarah can anticipate short-term relief from her life stress and reduction of her internal distress by binging. She has learned the soothing effects of food, the satiety and satisfaction that come from overeating. Food provides a reward, an escape from life's tensions. As the unhealthy choice is rewarded, she is not motivated to develop more functional, long-term solutions to her situational problems.

Stage 4—Short-Term Relief: As Sarah enters this stage, she experiences a reduction in negative thoughts, her tension is minimized, and her life seems better—for the moment. Guilt can also occur after relapsing into a behavior that you promised yourself or someone else you would avoid. Without long-term problem-solving skills, however, this motivated cycle will repeat again. Overeating can't stave off her emotional pain or her frustration with herself indefinitely. It is nothing more than short-term relief without any long-term resolution. In fact, the guilt, shame, and self-contempt that Sara experiences after overeating will likely propel her back to the beginning of the cycle.

Breaking the Cycle: Three Ways to Move From Compulsion To Real Emotional Change

Think about a repeated behavior you favor, one that causes your loved ones or good friends ask you, "Why do you do that?" The real answer, which you probably don't articulate, is that it relieves your emotional pain. It's a psychological anesthetic, but unfortunately, it wears off quickly and you build up a tolerance to its effect. For this reason, consider three alternatives to changing your emotions without resorting to compulsive behaviors. No doubt, Sarah doesn't see or want to consider alternatives to food, at least not initially. Because plowing through a bag of chips or eating a carton of ice cream helps her change from sad to happy, Sarah isn't interested in another approach. Of course, when she gains 100 pounds and everyone is pestering her to stop overeating and warning her that she's unattractive, unhealthy, and so on, she has greater motivation to try something else. You don't have to let yourself reach this stage, however. Instead, you can deal with your compulsions as early as possible by changing your feelings through one or more of these three alternatives: biochemical means, the sensorimotor system, and the cognitive processes.

Biochemical

It is hardly news that we can change how we feel by ingesting a chemical. We live in a culture that emphasizes life with no pain or discomfort. Over-the-counter medications exist for all that ails us. Manufacturers advertise quick relief. We no longer find any discomfort reasonable. Take this little pill, and all our problems will disappear. Commercials and advertisements bombard us with the mindset of perfection and the entitlement to instant relief. Popular mood changers include central nervous system depressants (alcohol, Xanex), antidepressants (Prozac, Lexapro), and narcotics (morphine and codeine). It is well-documented that biochemical interventions can be extremely effective and are often the quickest way to change emotions. They are often clinically necessary and quite helpful. Those suffering from bipolar disorder, for example, are routinely prescribed a treatment regimen that includes mood-stabilizing medications. It is only the abuse of chemicals that presents a problem.

However, the reality is that whenever we turn to an external source for problem solving, we develop a mindset that we are incapable of achieving the desired outcome without the external direction. In so doing, we teach ourselves to be less resourceful, less adaptive, and less able to productively impact our lives. So although a biochemical approach can be appropriate in certain conditions, it has serious drawbacks that you should consider carefully. Sarah can choose to take diet pills to control her overeating, but this may be no better a solution than overeating. She has just transferred her dependence from food to pills, and hasn't dealt effectively with the emotion underlying her compulsion. Our belief is that, in most cases, biochemical intervention should not be the first treatment of choice; behavioral approaches should be tried first. It is only when conditions are severe and unresponsive to other approaches that medication should be prescribed.

Sensorimotor

Another way to change feelings is through the sensorimotor system. That is, we can laugh, cry, run, jump, scream, or just relax to create an emotional change. This is very effective when used properly. A good cry can be highly cathartic when dealing with feelings of hurt and sadness. For example, Sarah has learned to express, through tears, her pain from the hurt she harbors as a result of being physically violated as a girl. The release of suppressed emotions has the power to change recurrent feelings of shame and inadequacy. In an effort to lose some of her excess weight, Sarah engages in brisk walking or swimming, activities that alter her emotional state not only because they help her lose weight but because they create a sense of power, control, and well-being (via endorphins). Another example of changing emotions through the sensorimotor system is listening to a relaxation tape to quell anxiety. This can also be accomplished through meditation, prayer, or yoga.

For years, we have been aware of the benefits of expressing emotions by saying them aloud to a trusted relative, friend, or therapist. There is research to support this. In a 2003 study published in *Science*, psychologist Dr. Matthew Leiberman found that verbalizing an emotion actually changes brain activity and reduces emotional pain and distress! If you've ever expressed your feelings, you may have amplified them in some way. When you talked about how your father made you feel ashamed when you were a child, you may have also found yourself shouting, punching the wall, crying, or doing any number of other things to magnify or dramatize your expression. Screaming or crying or smashing your fist into the wall may feel scary because you're losing control of your behavior, but it can also provide a sense of relief and empowerment. But be careful if you find yourself constantly amplifying your emotions in this manner. When you scream at your child to stop picking on his baby brother, you may get him to obey, but you also aren't dealing with your own feelings of inadequacy and frustration as a parent, and you may create a bad parent-child dynamic (your child obeys only when you scream). And if you start hitting things when you vent your emotions, you could hurt yourself or others.

Using your sensorimotor system to change your emotions is something we're all capable of doing productively, but you have to find the right method to express yourself. Take a cue from Jill, an 11-year-old girl who was severely anxious. Attempting to relieve her anxiety, she discovered that when she started bouncing on a back yard trampoline, her concerns diminished. The repetitive jumping stimulated the same endorphin release achieved by running, swimming, or any other aerobic activity. Physical exercise has been demonstrated to reduce symptoms of anxiety and depression. For some people with long-term depression or anxiety, exercise might not be the only approach used. Our point, though, is that you shouldn't underestimate the therapeutic potential of the sensorimotor system.

Cognition

Let's look at two different ways you can use your thoughts to change your feelings. First, you can adjust your mindset. This isn't as radical a move as revamping your entire perspective on a situation. Rather, it involves "changing the channel" in your head, shifting your focus from one issue to another. If you're neurotic about your love life—always doubting your ability to find someone and feeling tongue-tied and awkward when you go on a date—you don't suddenly have to start thinking of yourself as God's gift to womankind. Such a radical change of perspective is unrealistic and likely ineffectual. A mindset shift, on the other hand, is simply a move away from your usual obsessive thoughts, even if this shift is only for a brief time. When you make this adjustment, you often feel much different—and much better.

For instance, Jim is a mid-level manager with a large corporation who complains constantly about how he isn't appreciated by his bosses. When Jim was passed over for a promotion recently, he engaged in this compulsive complaining frequently and felt sorrier for himself than usual. At work, he took every opportunity to whine to trusted colleagues about this injustice. At home, too, he often lapsed into self-pitying moods. At dinner one night, Jim was complaining bitterly to his wife about how unfair it was that he was passed over for the promotion when they heard a loud crash coming from his young daughter's room. Jim raced up the stairs and found her partially buried, albeit unharmed, beneath a bookcase. After pulling his little girl to safety, Jim became aware of how his feelings had gone through a series of transformations: from bitterness and self-pity to fear, to relief, to amusement at his daughter's giggle once she knew she wasn't hurt, and, finally, to gratitude that his daughter was okay. Jim returned to the kitchen table and told his wife he was sorry for whining and complaining. He had realized in the past couple of minutes that he had so much to be grateful for.

It's not that Jim now considered the coworker's promotion to be fair—he still felt badly about it. He had simply shifted how he viewed the situation. Having recognized how fortunate he was to have a healthy, wonderful daughter took the edge off his negative feelings. As his focus shifted to his daughter, his emotions followed suit. He was able to feel tremendously grateful rather than tremendously wronged. The lesson: where our focus goes, our energy and feelings are sure to follow. This is why psychologists always recommend taking a "time out" during a heated argument. Getting the focus away from how wrong the other person is and on to something else, whether it be a magazine article, a cartoon, or a load of wash, may afford us the opportunity to refocus and feel differently. This breaks the cycle of compulsive behaviors, providing an exit from the stressful feelings that spawn these behaviors.

You have numerous cognitive options to change your mindset and take a break from your compulsive patterns. If you're obsessively moody or depressed, consider a bike ride. If you're anxious all the time, it may help to have a conversation with a friend who has a more serious problem. If you're always feeling sorry for yourself, try watching a stand-up comedy routine. Change the focus and you'll change the feelings. You may not realize it, but you probably have followed this advice before. It's why you blast music in the car when you're stuck in traffic gridlock; it's why you shop after a perceived disappointment; it's why you hop on the Internet after a difficult visit with a family member. Intuitively, you know that if do something that changes the way you're thinking, you'll impact your emotional state—and your behavior—for the better.

Although changing your mindset works in the short-term, the long-term method, which involves changing your emotional obsessions and moving away from unhealthy thinking patterns, is much more effective. Sarah's perception of herself includes the following: *I am a worthless person who can be used, violated, and taken advantage of by people if they so choose. I was not protected by my family because I am not important enough to care about. I will never amount to anything. I will not aspire to anything because I don't have the worth or the ability to pursue goals of any value. I am fat and undesirable, and people do not want me around. In order to keep the few people I have in my life, I must allow them to do what-ever it is they would like to do, even if they take advantage of me. There is no need to take care of my body or look attractive because to do so would only lead to more abuse from men. After all, I am not worth loving—only using and discarding.* This way of thinking imprisons Sarah in compulsive over-eating. It is theoretically impossible for her to change her core emotions (depression, self-pity) until she breaks free from the thinking patterns just described. While a mindset shift may help free her from her feelings in the short term, the odds are that she'll lapse back into them at some point in the future.

Sarah must practice fresh thinking and practice believing these new thoughts. She has to focus her mind on thoughts such as: I am a person of value and worth. My life is meaningful and worthwhile. I am capable of healing from the abuse of my childhood. The abuse was shameful; I am not. My children need a stable, loving parent; I am capable of being that parent. I do not need to be perfect. I am loving, kind, and responsible. I know this sounds disturbingly similar to an old Saturday Night Live skit on affirmations with a character named Stuart Smalley. "I am good enough; I'm smart enough; and, doggone it, people like me!" Beneath the satire, however, there is this Truth. You can teach yourself to think differently if you make a concerted effort to adopt and practice new thoughts. Or as they say in the AA program, "Fake it 'till you make it."

Albert Bandura, a psychologist and social cognitive theorist, coined the term *self-efficacy*, which provides insight into how we might use thoughts to change our behaviors. Bandura suggested that self-efficacy is both knowing that a given behavior produces a desired outcome, and possessing or having access to this behavior. Therefore, you may know that you need to stop fighting with your spouse all the time, but if you don't own this behavior cognitively, you'll be stuck. *Cognitive restructuring*, or changing what you tell yourself, allows you to own this behavior. This means that you catch yourself when you're using negative self-talk (*she deserves to be yelled at because she's wrong*) and substitute positive self-talk in its place (*I need to talk with her calmly and constructively*).

Shifting your thought and belief patterns can have an almost magical effect on your feelings. I (Chris) saw this in action when I was in graduate school. I observed a stage hypnotist invite dozens of people on stage and attempt to induce a trance in each of the volunteers. Those who fell into a trance were allowed to remain on stage; the rest were sent back to their seats. Once the hypnotist was confident in the suggestibility (compliance) of the volunteers, he began to play with their beliefs and perceptions of reality. For instance, he asked which of the volunteers came to the show with a spouse or date. He then said at the count of three, those volunteers would go into the audience, find their partners, and kiss them passionately. They did so. When he brought them back on stage and counted to three, he told them they would remember the kiss but believe it had taken place with a total stranger! I'll never forget the look of terror on the faces of two women subjects on that stage, one of them tearfully explaining, "My husband is going to kill me! I didn't even know that guy!" The hypnotist quickly corrected her perception, and the tears melted into smiles and laughter.

Let's return to Sarah. She sought treatment to deal with her many emotional and behavioral problems and symptoms, using all three approaches to break the hold of compulsive overeating and change her feelings about herself. Sarah has been taking an antidepressant. She has learned to express the emotional pain specific to her childhood hell. She has also taken up exercise and relaxation techniques. I encouraged her to meditate and pray to change her feelings, as well. Finally, Sarah has worked hard to move away from her irrational thought patterns (and accompanying beliefs and attitudes) that have held sway over her since she was a child. While Sarah is not yet at a place where she is totally free of her compulsive behaviors, she has made great progress in that direction, especially because she has learned that she is a valuable, responsible person, and has made a consistent effort to think and behave like one.

Diving Beneath the Surface

The ways in which people change compulsive behaviors varies. Statistics indicate that more than 90 percent of people who have quit smoking have done it on their own—no program, no clinician, no professional help. Others only stop their compulsive behavior when they acknowledge to themselves that they have a problem and seek programs to assist them. The best-known program, Alcoholics Anonymous, emphasizes a one-day-at-a-time approach to changing behavior, thoughts, and many other facets of living. The 12-step approach has been appropriated for the treatment of many other compulsive behaviors and addictions, including Gambler's Anonymous, Cocaine Anonymous, and even Sex and Love Addicts Anonymous. Other programs require the assistance of a therapist or coach.

Whether you choose to address your behaviors on your own or enlist the help of others, you're going to have to address the underlying emotional issues. This Truth is about changing your thinking *and* addressing your core emotional issues. Both actions are necessary to deal effectively with compulsions. When you shift your thinking patterns, you're going to bring buried emotional issues to the surface, and when you do so, you must confront them. Sarah, for instance, had to deal with traumatic emotional childhood issues and resolve them successfully to give herself the optimal chance of changing her relationship with food. In Sarah's quest to heal from her painful childhood memories, she discovered three underlying emotional states that triggered her compulsive behaviors: shame, fear, and resentment. These emotional states may have been born out of negative childhood experiences, including neglect and/or verbal, sexual, and physical abuse, and reemerged later in Sarah's life as a result of traumas, disappointments, repeated failures, and rejections.

Shame is the pervasive belief and feeling that you are bad or unworthy. It is consistently a product of abuse, especially sexual. The child internalizes the message, "You deserve to be treated badly because you are bad." If I believe I am bad, then it is much easier to justify overeating, smoking, or taking dangerous drugs because I am only hurting a bad person. It's the same attitude drivers have when driving an old, battered car: It's not a big deal to get one more scratch in the paint.

Fear lends itself to compulsive behaviors because it offers an escape from facing a feared object or situation head on. Although fear is an appropriate emotion for many situations, it can become a toxic reflex for dealing with myriad life situations. If you think of yourself as weak and inadequate, you will approach life with a predictable response of fear and anxiety. To replace fear with a healthy self-confidence, we must believe in the possibility that life can be different, that change is possible. Then we must bravely face long-standing fears and conquer them one by one. New thinking must replace established beliefs that feature self-doubt, inadequacy, and potential catastrophe.

Resentment is the cornerstone of compulsive behaviors. According to some experts, it is the number-one reason that recovering alcoholics relapse. This emotional state has also been linked to heart disease, strokes, depression, and anxiety. The resentful individual medicates his or her anger and hatred with a mood-changing compulsion that only temporarily assuages the pain. Shopping, TV-watching, gossiping, and obsessive exercising can all afford temporary relief from the intensity of that resentment and dull the emotional pain. On the other hand, some compulsions, such as drinking, serve to fuel the fire of resentment and may engender a dangerous combination of rage and lack of inhibition.

Despite the temporary balm compulsive behaviors may provide, these powerful underlying emotions will surface again, and you'll need to increase the intensity and frequency of your compulsion in order to deal with them. It's an escalating game you're bound to lose. At some point, your emotional hurt will be too great to mask with any behavior. You can't ignore these underlying emotions. Therefore, figure out what emotions are fueling your compulsions and address them. For instance, Mary discovered a pocket of resentment when she quit smoking cigarettes. She experienced angry feelings toward her husband—feelings that she had hidden from both herself and him in clouds of smoke for the past 35 years! To remain smoke free, she required a plan that included understanding, expressing, and releasing her resentment and anger. Once she addressed the stuffed emotions, she was no longer imprisoned by the counterproductive, obsessive feelings and thoughts or the compulsive behaviors.

Now let's focus on some exercises that will help you change your thoughts and concomitant feelings in order to change your compulsive behaviors.

Exercises

In this chapter, you learned about the connection between thoughts, feelings, and beliefs and behaviors. You also learned that emotions impact your life in different ways. Emotions can move you forward in a healthy and productive direction, or they can overwhelm you and cause you to make unwise choices and decisions.

Exercise 1—Take a Poll

Identify supportive family members and friends and ask them to provide input regarding your counterproductive behaviors. As you'll see, the following form refers to these behaviors in three different ways—a loved one may not consider your constant TV- watching to be a compulsion but he or she may label it as an unhealthy habit. Some of you may be aware of your compulsive behaviors, but many of you may have rationalized them as harmless activities. This poll will alert you about the behaviors you may need to work on.

Name _____

Compulsive Behavior _____

    Suggestion _____

_____

Name _____

Unhealthy Habit _____

    Suggestion _____

    _____

Name _____

Area to Work on _____

    Suggestion _____

    _____

Exercise 2—The Relapse Monitor

This activity is designed to help you monitor the thoughts and emotions that lead to relapses. You may successfully stop or moderate your compulsive behavior, but over time, you rationalize the return to this behavior. Use this monitor to watch for the pivotal point at which your resolve disappears and the compulsion resumes:

1. What is the problem behavior you want to change?

    _____

    _____

    _____

2. Write out your constructive internal dialogue when you avoid the undesirable behavior.

    _____

    _____

    _____

3. Describe the times when you have returned to the negative behavior.

    _____

_____

_____

4. What events occurred between abstinence and relapse?

_____

_____

_____

5. List the triggers for your relapses, for example, people, places, stress, internal dialogue, changing focus from negative impact to reward.

_____

_____

_____

6. What emotions have contributed to your previous relapses?

_____

_____

_____

7. Compare the rewards of the undesirable behavior you want to change and the desirable behavior you want to establish.

_____

_____

_____

Exercise 3—The Change-Your-Thoughts Practice

We realize that changing your thought patterns can be a challenge.

You've been thinking one way for years, so to switch that pattern after all that time requires great focus. More than that, it requires practice. Here, we've designed a simple exercise to help you practice catching yourself thinking the wrong way. As you'll see, we want you to work at raising your awareness of the link between negative-self talk and compulsive behaviors, and then fashion a positive statement to yourself to substitute for the negative one. Do this often enough, and it will become second nature.

Situation _____

    Unproductive behavior _____

    Negative self-talk _____

    Alternative positive statement to self _____

    _____

Situation _____

    Unproductive behavior _____

    Negative self-talk _____

    Alternative positive statement to self _____

    _____

Situation _____

    Unproductive behavior _____

    Negative self-talk _____

    Alternative positive statement to self _____

    _____

Situation _____

    Unproductive behavior _____

Negative self-talk _____

Alternative positive statement to self _____

Exercise 4—Break the Cycle

You may have developed repetitive behaviors or compulsions that provide short-term relief from negative feelings. They reduce your tension but do not resolve the cause. In this exercise, we provide a plan to halt the cycle of obsessive thoughts and compulsive behavior. By bringing this unconscious process to light, you will become more aware of your patterns and responsive, rather than reactive, to stressful situations. By recording your impulsive thoughts and subsequent behaviors, your heightened awareness may break the cycle of compulsive behaviors.

Step 1: For one week, list the times when you have an intrusive obsessive thought. Also record the subsequent behavior and the time lag between the two.

Step 2: After one week increase your reaction time. Your goal is to delay impulsive reaction to the thought so that eventually you will be able to substitute a more planned response. You may not yet be able to keep obsessive thoughts out of your head, but your subsequent behavior is within your control.

Step 3: Continue to increase the time between your idea and your behavior each week until you feel comfortable that you are responding constructively rather than impulsively.

	Sun	Mon	Tues	Wed	Thurs	Fri	Sat
Thought							
Behavior							
Alternative							
Thought							
Behavior							
Alternative							
Thought							
Behavior							
Alternative							
Thought							
Behavior							
Alternative							
Thought							
Behavior							
Alternative							

Chapter 3

Every Behavior Has an Underlying Purpose, and It's Not Always What We Think

I don't get upset over things I can't control because if I can't control them, there's no use getting upset. And I don't get upset over things I can control because if I can control them, what's the use in getting upset?

—Mickey Rivers,
former New York Yankee

Faith ends where worry begins. Worry ends where faith begins.

—Anonymous

Ruth was 64 when she developed a curious habit in the last year of her life: shopping. Although shopping is a common habit, her style of shopping concerned her and ultimately led her to treatment. Ruth spent hours at the mall buying hundreds of dollars of clothing only to return most or all of it within a few days. Ruth was aware that her behavior wasn't normal, but she was driven to repeat it without any conscious awareness of her actions. Insight alone is not necessarily curative, but she needed to understand her behavior before she could do anything about it. Ruth's behavior was meeting a need or she wouldn't engage in it. The Truth here is that behavior is purposeful, and identifying that purpose can liberate you to behave in a more authentic, productive manner.

What was Ruth's purpose for her admittedly strange form of shopping? We'll examine Ruth's motivation in the next section, but for now, consider the following questions:

- ▶ Why would a teenager grab a sharpened blade, cut herself on her upper arm where no one could see it, and watch the blood drip?

- ▶ Why would a man spend an hour channel surfing, never stopping more than a minute to watch any one television program?

- ▶ Why would a mother nag her children when she is well aware that it provokes and frustrates them?

- ▶ Why would a man thirsting for love and intimacy keep all of his relationships at arm's length?

- ▶ Why would a woman keep her husband's ashes in a box on her bureau and hold one-sided conversations with it for as long as an hour at a time?

- ▶ Why would a baseball player wear the same unwashed, smelly T-shirt under his uniform every game for years?

Each behavior meets a need for each of these individuals, even though the need may seem bizarre. For instance, many young women engage in cutting themselves because it provides a physical release for emotional pain. It is not coincidental that the one controlling the pain is the victim herself who directs where, when, and how she will inflict her wounds. The external pain purges her inner feelings, giving her a sense of release and relief. Because the cutting provides her with the relief she craves, a young woman is likely to repeat the behavior. Behavior that does not meet a need will die; only behavior that serves a purpose survives.

Some purposes are relatively easy to understand. The baseball player wears the ratty T-shirt as a good luck charm. Channel surfing provides some people with a buzz, relieving boredom and providing a sense of excitement. Logically, these purposes may not stand up under scrutiny, but they meet real needs, no matter how illogical they might seem to an outside observer. If a behavior is not reinforced, it tends to die (in behavioral terms, it is *extinguished*). Consequently, all behavior makes sense to us on some level at the time we are engaging in it or we would not do it. This does not mean that we always understand the particular need the behavior is meeting; we may only know that we have to do it.

Purposeful Misbehavior

Consider the purpose of lying. We lie when we are afraid of the consequences of telling the truth; or, as University of Massachusetts psychologist Dr. Robert Feldman suggests, "It's tied in with self-esteem. We find that as people feel that their self-esteem is threatened, they immediately begin to lie at higher levels" (*Journal of Basic and Applied Psychology*, 2006). Our colleague, Dr. Jill Scarpellini, tells this story about the purposefulness of lying and the time of life when this behavior usually first appears. She walked into the room where her 2-year-old, David, had been playing alone for about five minutes. Books and toys were strewn everywhere. Jill was a bit startled by the transformation that had taken place in what had been a neat and organized room. The perceptive David caught his mother's eye and described the room in a word—"Mess!" Ever the psychologist, Jill responded to David by asking the question, "How do you suppose it got that way?" David paused a moment to search for the best possible answer. "Grandpa," he replied.

Now think about why people gossip. Passing on rumors and innuendos about people raises our status in a group by providing interesting, compelling information about others not present. As Dr. Marion Underwood, author of *Social Aggression Among Girls*, points out, gossiping can also be "an effective way to be aggressive [to other girls] without facing social sanctions."

Marital infidelity, too, has a purpose beyond physical pleasure. Although statistics vary significantly regarding the number of unfaithful spouses, Janice Cable, in an article in the August/September 2005 issue of *Industry* magazine, titled "Our Cheatin' Hearts: Infidelity: How to Stop Before You Start," cites the following information on the prevalence and causes of marital infidelity: 22 percent of married men and 14 percent of married women have had affairs at least once during their married lives.

She states, "People cheat to replace some emotional component that they aren't getting in the relationship—whether it's intimacy, attention, seduction, or a combination. People also cheat because they are bored or angry or lost. These reasons apply equally to men and women."

Alfred Adler, an internationally renowned psychiatrist and student of Freud, postulated that children misbehave for one of four reasons: to seek attention, to gain control/power, to exact revenge, or to display inadequacy. Usually the child is not consciously aware of these goals, but a parent would do well to understand what motivates the child's misbehavior in order to respond most appropriately.

As you can see, what you see is not always what you get. Behavior is never random, nor is the purpose of that behavior always obvious. Just as children may not realize they are acting like spoiled brats because they crave attention, adults may not understand that they're gossiping in order to earn status in a group.

So what about Ruth? What could she possibly derive from her self-defeating cycle of buying and exchanging? First, you should know that Ruth had recently been rejected sexually by her husband. The rebuff was so painful that she began to avoid him as much as possible. As part of her avoidance, she spent a lot of time outside the home, which included shopping expeditions to the mall. There, she discovered several nice saleswomen. Ruth enjoyed their companionship sometimes for hours on end. The attention and the compliments she received when she tried on dresses were gratifying, and helped her to combat some of the negative perceptions of herself that she had been entertaining since her husband's rejection. Unfortunately, after she got home and realized what she had purchased and how much she had spent, Ruth knew she neither needed all of the clothes nor could she afford to make these kinds of purchases. She would go back to the store when she knew she wouldn't run into the same salesladies and return the majority of her purchases.

Because of her husband's rejection, Ruth experienced powerful feelings of rejection and inadequacy. Whenever these feelings descended on her, she would run to the mall where she would receive compliments and avoid being in her husband's presence as well as the environment that acted as a trigger for those hurtful feelings. Understanding the purpose of Ruth's behavior leads back to the importance of her dealing with her relationship with her husband. The feelings of rejection and inadequacy that she harbored were now being used to fuel her new shopping habit. As soon as Ruth felt these uncomfortable emotions, she experienced an urge to make a beeline to the mall. By doing so, she avoided her discomfort for another day.

Avoidance Feels Good Now But Not Later

Avoidance is a common behavioral purpose, and it does provide short-term relief. That's why people like Ruth act the way they do—their behaviors help them avoid confronting troubling situations and unpleasant emotions. What avoidance doesn't do, however, is help them resolve the underlying problem. Because Ruth's escapist behavior did not address her marital conflict, it could not resolve it. Hence, the unhealthy cycle of conflict and avoidance resulted in serial shopping.

Unless you really examine your behavior closely and deeply, you may not realize your purpose is avoidance. Ruth could have found 100 reasons to justify her shopping—it got her out of the house, she got to meet new people, she loved to try on clothes—but she could have easily missed how its purpose was avoidance. We just aren't used to thinking in these terms, and as a consequence, we blithely continue with our reflexive and often counterproductive behaviors.

Part of the problem is that avoidance makes no logical sense in many situations, so we don't see it as the motivator for what we do—or for what others do, for that matter. A friend was disappointed by the fact that he could not seem to get a return phone call from someone from whom he had requested a job. "I don't get it," he complained. "Isn't it common courtesy to call back and tell me he doesn't have a job to offer me?" Courtesy? Yes. Common? Maybe not. The prospective employer probably didn't return the call because he didn't want to feel uncomfortable. Who wants to be the bearer of bad tidings? Who wants to dash someone's hopes? Where there's discomfort, there's often avoidance. People will often choose the path of least resistance, which usually means avoiding anything that appears to be scary, painful, or even mildly uncomfortable. That's why we put off the breakup, the spring cleaning, or the colonoscopy. Avoidance leads to relief, which is preferable to the unpleasant alternatives.

An Emotional Purpose: An Unwillingness to Let Go of Feelings

Some of us act the way we do because we don't want to let go of certain feelings—not just good feelings, such as joy or pride, but feelings that most of us would classify as negative: resentment, bitterness, fear, worry, and anger. We do so because we receive physiological and psychological payoffs from these feelings.

Anger and resentment, for instance, may seem like things everyone wants to get rid of, but they serve a purpose. If we release our anger, we become 100-percent responsible for our happiness and success. When we store up that anger or resentment, we make sure that we don't take responsibility for what is making us unhappy; in fact, we may transfer that responsibility to another person or an institution. For instance, Dave is a war veteran who is angry at his country for treatment he received both in Southeast Asia and upon his return stateside. Despite the fact that he has been home for more than 25 years, he reminds himself daily of how he was victimized. His anger is purposeful. He believes if he releases it, he will condone the unfair way he was treated and, in effect, will have joined the side of the enemy, the U.S. government. Dave also clings to his anger because he doesn't want to take responsibility for his own happiness and success, a disturbing prospect after so many years of under-functioning in isolation and contempt. Of course, Dave doesn't look at his anger, this way. He doesn't understand its purpose. To him, anger and resentment have become conditioned reflexes, appropriate responses to the "wrongs" done to him.

People hold on to their emotions for other reasons, including the perception that accepting the reality of a situation means accepting defeat. Michael stayed angry at his estranged brother for 30 years. Although Michael can barely remember the fight they had years ago, he keeps his anger toward his brother because forgiveness would mean he was admitting weakness, and that he was wrong and his brother was right. Hence, this way of thinking maintains his anger toward and estrangement from his only remaining family member. Michael's anger is meeting a need, so he continues to feed it. Again, Michael might maintain that the reason he's angry is because his brother is a jerk; it would be all about what's wrong with his brother rather than the payoff he gets for being angry.

Self-protection is another reason we don't let go of emotions. When we stop being angry or resentful, we believe we're making ourselves vulnerable. For example, Jane has been divorced twice; in both instances, her husbands cheated on her. She was mad at her first husband and even angrier at her second one, and Jane has been clinging to that fury ever since. As a result, she hasn't had a meaningful relationship in five years; the anger and bitterness spoil every relationship as soon as things start to get serious. Jane prefers to seek safety in her anger than allow any man to hurt her as her first two husbands did.

Here's one more purpose emotional clinging serves: maintaining power and control or the upper hand. This is an especially common purpose for anger, as Mrs. Wilson demonstrates. Mrs. Wilson tends to intimidate the students in her classroom. She seems to enjoy making a big deal out of mistakes made by her young cosmetology students. It appears to the students that she derives pleasure out of exploiting their imperfections and lack of experience. Mrs. Wilson has no friends. Her life is her work. She was sexually abused as a little girl, never married, and has never allowed anyone to get close to her. Her fear of being violated or hurt in any way has translated into a decision to be angry and hostile. In this way, she always has the upper hand. As the teacher, Mrs. Wilson is in a superior position to her students, allowing her to be the perpetrator rather than the victim.

We've focused our discussion primarily on anger since it's such a common emotion that people hold on to, but people cling to a wide variety of other emotions. Denise has wallowed in sadness over her sister's death for 12 years. Being sad at the death of a sibling is perfectly normal and healthy, but when it dominates one's emotional state and continues beyond a reasonable time frame, something else is going on. Denise discovered that holding on to that sadness was her way of keeping her late sister alive. She fears that she will lose touch with that cherished relationship if she allows her sadness to dissipate. In her own mind, Denise thinks that being sad is the least she can do to honor the memory of her sister. She doesn't realize that holding tight to this emotional teddy bear prevents her from enjoying her relationships with other family and friends or taking pleasure in her hobbies. The whole purpose of her sadness is to defy nature and keep her sister alive. To demonstrate that she cares so much about her sister, she won't ever be happy again.

Like anger and sadness, fear can also have us in its grip. As we mentioned in Chapter 1, fear is a feeling state that reminds us of a perceived threat or danger. Once we receive that message, fear has served its purpose and is not necessary to maintain. Many people live their lives in fear and/or anxiety because it helps them avoid things that are unpleasant or potentially threatening to their self-esteem. Avoidance of a potentially threatening situation accomplishes two things: it provides immediate relief, and it increases the fear the next time that specific situation or stimulus is introduced. Let's say you're afraid of flying. A friend tells you about fabulous trip he has planned to a place you always wanted to visit, and he invites you to join him. As much as you want to go, you turn him down, making an excuse that it costs too much or lying that you never had much interest in that particular place. On the surface, clinging to your fear of flying seems nonsensical; but as soon as you turn your friend down, you experience this huge feeling of relief. The next time you're tempted to fly you'll feel even more afraid, which ensures that you will again avoid dealing with your fear, which means you'll again experience that sweet relief.

Whatever fear we cling to and whatever behavior this emotional clinging engenders, the behavior tends to escalate over time. You may have been somewhat awkward and hesitant when you turned down your friend's offer of a wonderful trip. Next time, however, you will be a bit smoother in your excuse-making and more credible in your tone of voice and body language. In short, you become more skilled in the art of avoidance. You never resolve the deeper problem, because your behavior is purposeful—it allows you to maintain your particular negative emotion. And the thing of it is, you remain beset with your fears and anxieties. You many never fly on a plane for the rest of your life, but you remain terrified at even the thought of going on a plane.

Henrietta lives her life frightened of every potential social encounter. Her perception of herself as inadequate and unlovable is central to her way of looking at the world, and she holds fast to her fear of every social contact. Even when an opportunity presents itself (such as an invitation to a party or a male showing interest in her), she returns to her fear to provide sufficient justification to avoid what might be a fun and rewarding interaction. Why? Because she could get hurt or rejected or humiliated or embarrassed! Consequently, living in fear allows her to escape from any potentially dangerous situation. Keeping her fear is self-protective. At the same time, it reinforces her conclusion that she is inadequate and unlovable. From Henrietta's skewed perspective, maintaining her fear makes sense. Without addressing her fear and the underlying purpose it serves, Henrietta can never develop the interpersonal skills needed to foster a healthy relationship or to establish healthy boundaries. Unfortunately, her understanding of intimate relationships remains limited. She may continue to enter into relationships where she's hurt—emotionally or physically—and which confirm her belief that the world is a dangerous place and relationships must be avoided.

Guilt is another feeling that people hold onto long after it has proven to be useful. Guilt is a reminder that we have betrayed our own moral code. It's a good thing to feel guilt, because a society that feels no guilt is a dangerous place; sociopaths feel no remorse after killing someone. Yet to harbor guilt long after receiving its message is self-destructive. Why would we hold onto guilt? Because by staying in guilt and wallowing in the accompanying shame, we can justify underachieving and avoid challenges and responsibilities. It is easier to continue to remind ourselves that we are bad, undeserving, and inadequate than it is to address and change these beliefs. As with anger, people tend to stay stuck in guilt rather than take responsibility for being happy and successful.

There are factors from our family of origin that may also contribute to the development and persistence of guilt feelings. If we habitually react with guilt in relationships, it could be that we were taught early in life that we were responsible for how others feel. In childhood, we became convinced that our behaviors controlled others' reactions. When people cling to guilt, they usually possess low self-esteem and blame themselves when things go wrong. We go through life telling ourselves, *How bad of me, I am at fault*, and *If I hadn't done x, y, or z, things would be different.* We assume responsibility for all the negatives that occur to others. This grandiose delusion serves the purpose of keeping our guilt intact. As long as we believe that we're responsible for everything bad that happens, we will always feel guilty.

Don't fret—we didn't forget chronic worrying

What purpose does worrying serve? Who wants anxiety and insomnia? Many people will tell you that they hate to worry all the time, but that they just can't help it. In *The Worry Cure: Seven Steps to Stopping Worrying*, Dr. Robert Leahy claims that 38 percent of the population can be classified as chronic worriers. These are the people you can walk up to any time of the day or night and ask, "What are you worried about?" and there will always be an answer, because as long as they are awake they are worrying.

You can control your worrying, but you must understand that it serves a very clear purpose: keeping you in touch with a situation that is otherwise outside of your control. When you don't worry, you give up control. Most psychologists understand that people prefer having control over a situation rather than admitting to complete powerlessness and vulnerability. Consequently, worry is a mental strategy, albeit an unconscious one, that makes us feel as if we can influence a situation over which we may have no influence at all. The parent who anxiously paces when her children are on an airplane to return to college after spring break is attempting to maintain some degree of control over the success of the flight and the safety of her children. If she relaxed and stopped worrying, she would be admitting that she is vulnerable and powerless. She prefers to watch the weather channel and stay off the telephone waiting to hear from her children, with images of plane crashes in her head. When the children finally arrive safely at college and call to let mom know that everything is okay, the worrying mother feels a great sense of relief. If she is honest enough to admit it, she may also feel a sense of accomplishment at having successfully worried them back to their dorm rooms. This experience reinforces her worrying behavior. The next time she feels powerless and is emotionally invested in an outcome, she'll repeat her worrying ritual. The apparent payoff: worrying about something seems to increase the odds that what she's worrying about won't happen.

Worry is a superstitious behavior. Think about the football fan who must sit in a certain chair, wearing the same old hat backward, when rooting for his beloved team each Sunday afternoon. On some level, he is rational enough to be aware that his behavior is unlikely to affect the outcome of the contest, but he enjoys the illusion of control, the sense that his ritual is having a positive impact in some vague way. It's also instructive to consider when this football fan's ritual began. A few years ago, his team was losing by 21 points in the fourth quarter when they made a miraculous comeback and won the game. When this happened, this fan was sitting in that lucky chair with that lucky hat on backward. The reinforcement of those behaviors leads him to conclude that this is what he must do from now on to have some control over his team's performance.

Remember, too, that our Truth states that people often don't know the purpose behind their behaviors, and this football fan is no exception. If you were to ask him about why he engages in his Sunday afternoon ritual during games, he would laugh and tell you it's just a silly superstition. Or he might respond seriously and say that although he knows there probably isn't any connection between the ritual and winning, the team has won seven straight so why risk changing the routine. What he won't say is that these worrying rituals give him a sense of control over the game's outcome.

The problem with worrying rituals is that they can result in extreme behaviors. For instance, Sam was a sports junkie, the quintessential rabid fan. While watching a football game wherein his beloved team was trailing by a touchdown in the third quarter, his wife foolishly decided to use the bathroom. Her decision was foolish because her husband's team scored two touchdowns while she was gone. When her husband concluded that it was her bathroom visit that inspired his team's comeback, he locked his wife in the bathroom for the rest of the game! While this story is amusing, the consequences of worrying rituals are anything but. When people don't grasp the real purpose of their behaviors, they can fall into all sorts of routines that cause them to act in ways that alienate others. At their worst, these behaviors can destroy valued relationships.

A true "worry wart" always worries; if there isn't something in his life that produces anxiety and fretting, he'll create it. He tends to believe that he is the only one who truly "gets" the problem, and he must take the appropriate action of worrying to remedy it. On *Sesame Street*, Burt sees Ernie holding a banana in his ear and asks, "Why do you have a banana in your ear?" Ernie says, "It is to keep the elephants away." Burt responds, "There are no elephants here." Ernie proudly states, "See, it works."

Like other troublesome emotions such as fear and anger, worry will have an iron grip on our behavior until we understand its true purpose. To stop worrying we must admit to powerlessness and vulnerability. Ultimately, we must believe that whatever will be, will be okay. That is, the antidote to worry is faith. Faith may be in God, in fate, in self, or some combination thereof. Faith is the realization that because we are not in control, our worrying will not impact the outcome of the situation. We may view the world as being God's to control, and see ourselves as being in his great big hands (think of the Allstate ads); or perhaps our belief is that we are capable enough to negotiate life regardless of what happens. We may believe in the dictum of "what comes around goes around," so if we're good, good things will happen for us. Or we may believe that anything that is out of our control is out of our control, so why worry about it.

Perhaps you're aware of the serenity prayer: "God grant me the serenity to accept the things I cannot change, the courage to change the things I can, and the wisdom to know the difference." If you live your life trying to control things that are beyond your control, you're going to engage in rituals and routines that provide only temporary relief. Emotionally healthy people, on the other hand, may have all sorts of concerns and problems, but they're able to cope with them by accepting their lack of control and vulnerability in some areas, and then by finding something to believe in that provides comfort and context. Whether you pray for guidance or have faith in your own ability to muddle through worrisome situations, you have a good understanding of why you're doing what you're doing. When you have a point of view about life and why things happen, you have access to a larger purpose and don't have to resort to worrying to deal with scary situations.

Understanding purpose with a lowercase p

There's been a lot of talk recently about finding your Purpose-with-a-capital-p. The notion is that if you can figure out what why you are here, life will be more fulfilling and meaningful. But finding your larger Purpose can be a journey, one that takes a great deal of time and effort. Although this is a noble goal, the Truth in this book is focused more on small steps. As you begin to understand the purpose behind your anger or your anxiety or your sadness, you can start moving toward that larger Purpose. If you can figure out why you shop addictively or are in perpetual mourning or worry obsessively about things beyond your control, then you're that much closer to a happy, rewarding life. All this means you need to focus on what you get out of a particular behavior. What reward do you get from it? What payoff do you receive from wallowing in a negative emotion? To get at these answers, you need to ask yourself some tough questions about your fears:

▶ If you stop meddling in the business of your adult children, what is it you fear?

▶ If you let go of your long-standing anger toward your mother, ex-spouse, or former business partner, what do you fear would happen?

▶ If you finally give away your late husband's clothes, what consequences do you fear?

By understanding your fear, you can decide to overcome it, thus emerging from self-defeating patterns of behavior. By recognizing the irrational basis for your fear, you can glimpse the purpose of your old behaviors. The following exercises will assist you in understanding why you do what you do and how to change your behavior by changing your thinking.

Exercises

Exercise 1—Why Do You Bang Your Head Against the Wall?

To make use of this chapter's Truth, you need to figure out your behavior's true purpose. This first exercise will help you figure out why you engage in any behavior that has negative consequences. Think about a common, stressful situation you experience and how you act in this situation. Then answer the following questions:

1. What are your habits when you're dealing with this stressful event, person, or situation? What behaviors do you repeatedly engage in?

_____

_____

_____

2. What releases your pent-up emotions or feelings (for example, anxiety or guilt)?

_____

_____

_____

3. What behaviors do you exhibit that you have been told are unhealthy or that you should stop?

_____

_____

_____

Now for each identified behavior, answer the following questions:

1. What purpose does it serve?

_____

_____

_____

2. What are you avoiding when you engage in this behavior?

_____

_____

_____

3. Where did you learn this behavior?

_____

_____

_____

4. What skills do you need to develop (such as assertiveness, patience, organization, independence, or trust) to replace your negative behavior?

_____

_____

_____

Exercise 2—The Avoidance Identifier

If the previous exercise didn't help you figure out your counterproductive behavior and the purpose it serves, this one might. When your repeated behavior is designed to avoid a certain type of discomfort, it's a clue that there's a problem. The following is a list of five common situations that people avoid. Make a check next to the one that applies to you:

❑ Being confrontational.

❑ Being emotionally intimate.

❑ Sharing a personal weakness.

❑ Admitting you're at fault.

❑ Talking negatively about someone.

Now describe the particular behavioral routine you use to avoid experiencing a particular situation:

1. What are the common things you say to avoid this situation?

    _____

    _____

    _____

2. What are the common things you do to avoid this situation?

    _____

    _____

    _____

3. How does what you say or do help you avoid the situation that makes you uncomfortable?

    _____

    _____

    _____

Exercise 3—Name Your Favorite Unpleasant Emotion

Many times, our purpose in acting a certain way is to sustain one or more of the following emotions: anger, fear, worry, resentment, bitterness. Ask yourself the questions under each emotion to see which one applies to you.

Anger

1. Do you find yourself becoming furious at someone or some situation at least once a day?

2. Do you find yourself feeling good after being angry? Is there a sense of relief or satisfaction in the anger?

3. Do you rationalize/justify your anger to yourself without asking too many questions about why you're so angry?

4. Have other people told you that you have a bad temper and need to figure out why you're so furious so much of the time?

Fear

1. Is it is difficult for you to go through a day without feeling deeply fearful about something?

2. Though this fear may be scary in one sense, is it also oddly comforting in another sense? Do you crave that fearful sensation?

3. Do you often tell yourself that you have every right to be afraid without ever examining why you're so frightened?

4. Have others expressed concern to your about your fears and suggest that they're preventing you from doing something (establishing a new relationship, getting a job)?

Worry

1. Is it fair to describe you as a worry-wart?

2. What happens when you worry a lot? Is there a sense that worrying somehow prevents bad things from happening?

3. Do you frequently insist to yourself that you'd be crazy if you didn't worry about the things that occupy you?

4. Does your worrying interfere with getting things accomplished or maintaining good relationships? Do people tell you that you worry too much?

Resentment

1. Do you frequently engage in self-talk in which you feel sorry for yourself? Do you often tell others that you are the victim in a given scenario?

2. Does expressing your resentment make you feel good? Is talking about how you've been taken advantage of or passed over a way at striking back at those who have hurt you?

3. Do you often tell yourself that you have plenty to be resentful about? That it's not your fault that people don't understand you or are so mean or stupid?

4. Does your resentment turn off other people? Do they tell you that you have to stop acting like a victim and take charge of your life?

Bitterness

1. Do you often find yourself regretting the path your life has taken and feeling like you've made bad choices?

2. Is bitterness a soothing feeling in some ways? Do you keep replaying certain negative events in your mind to create that bitter taste?

3. Do you believe that being bitter is a perfectly logical reaction to the way things are? Do you find yourself unable to communicate well with others who don't share your feelings of bitterness?

4. Does your bitterness result in a certain amount of social isolation? Do you prefer to wallow in your bitterness rather than have fun and communicate with others?

Chapter 4

We All Sabotage Ourselves Unless We Confront Our Internal Saboteur

No doubt, you've known someone who acts in ways that are clearly not in his or her best interest. You may have a friend who confounds you and others because she says or does things that seem almost calculated to get her in trouble—often the same kind of trouble time after time. Maybe you yourself have done things that seem counterproductive or irrational. Even as you're making a bad choice, the logical part of your brain screams, *Don't do it!* What's going on? Consider Mike's story:

> In my junior year of college, I met a young lady, Suzie, who quite literally took my breath away. Suzie was adorably cute, very athletic—essentially everything I was looking for in a girlfriend. One Friday afternoon, I mustered the courage to ask Suzie out on a date and, much to my amazement, she said yes! I remember we went on a double date, but for the life of me, I can't remember who the other couple was because I was so smitten with Suzie. When I took her back to her dorm, we talked at least another hour and a half before we finally said goodnight. As far as I could tell, she had as much fun as I did. I returned to my dorm room floating on cloud nine with visions of a forever relationship dancing in my head. Then I never asked her out again! The school year ended, Suzie transferred to another college, and I never saw her again.

Why would Mike prohibit himself from pursuing someone with whom he believed he could be very happy? It makes absolutely no sense unless you understand the concept of the internal saboteur. Beneath the level of consciousness, something inside Mike whispered, *Mike, don't ask her out again. What if she says no? What if she says yes, you have an even better time, and then she dumps you? What if you're not worthy of her? It's too scary to even contemplate.* This subconscious whispering voice made Mike afraid to ask Suzie out; it raised the possibility that he could be rejected, and this was a terribly fearsome prospect for him. On a conscious level, Mike didn't understand why he failed to call Suzie. It didn't occur to him that he was sabotaging his own potential for joy and happiness because of his fear of rejection. As much as he liked Suzie, part of him liked avoiding rejection even more. It was only when Mike was in therapy that he learned about the saboteur—the internal voice that tried to protect him from imminent danger—and that this voice was responsible for his inertia. He also discovered that this wasn't the first time he'd "hired" this saboteur for what seemed like self-protection. The saboteur's chicanery had resulted in Mike's acting against his own best interests a number of times throughout his life.

The saboteur operates in the shadows of our subconscious. That's why Mike and most of the rest of us aren't aware of it and the damage it does. To make use of Truth # 4, we need to bring the saboteur out of the darkness and see it for what it really is.

Seems Like a Friend, Acts Like a Foe

To grasp this Truth, you need to get your mind around a psychological paradox: You may say you want one thing, but your actions reveal that you want something else. The following story illustrates this very well.

Two hardworking factory workers break for lunch on a busy Monday. They grab their lunch pails and tear into the plastic wrap to unveil the day's sandwiches. Worker One peeks underneath his bread and states in dismay, "Peanut butter. I hate peanut butter." Worker Two watches silently. Tuesday's lunch break reveals a similar scene, with Worker One again peeking under his bread to find the same sticky substance. "Peanut butter!" he exclaims, "I hate peanut butter." Worker Two again says nothing. On Wednesday, the same two workers break for lunch at the usual time. Worker One excitedly removes his sandwich from its wrapping. Carefully he lifts the bread to reveal the contents of today's sandwich. "Peanut butter!" he yells, pounding his fist on the break room table in frustration. "I hate peanut butter!" His buddy is now compelled to speak after watching the same scenario for three straight days. "Hey," he says. "I know this is none of my business, but why don't you tell your wife to make you some other sandwich besides peanut butter?" Worker One shoots a fiery glance at his coworker and says, "Hey, pal, leave my wife out of this. I make my own lunch!"

So it is with the saboteur, which is a self-created mind-set that protects the self from apparent danger. In the previous story, Worker One may have feared any break from his eating routine. Even though he couldn't stand the thought of another peanut butter sandwich for lunch, he preferred it to the unknown of tuna salad, smoked turkey or whatever else he might have substituted. Or rather, his saboteur was supposedly acting in his best interest, protecting him from the fearful unknown.

People grapple with many fears that provide opportunities to call upon the saboteur: rejection, failure, success, intimacy, and loss of control. We call on this fellow to defend ourselves from fear and situations that we perceive as overwhelming. When we lack confidence to negotiate a particular situation or relationship in our lives, we summon the saboteur. During therapy, Mike came to understand that if he was merely afraid that Suzie wouldn't grant him a second date, he probably would not have called upon his saboteur. His real fear, though, was much larger and deeper, based on his feeling that he was unworthy of such a lovely woman. It seemed to him inevitable that she would soon figure that out and reject him. His fear was that he could not handle the feelings of rejection. Rather than risk dealing with those emotions, his saboteur dealt with the problem by convincing Mike not to ask her out again.

Failure isn't the only fear that awakens the saboteur. Laura, a top volleyball player in her high school, unwittingly engaged her saboteur during her senior year. Passionate about the game, Laura won the MVP award at the annual sports banquet at the end of her junior year season. She was honored and excited initially, but when the weight of being the best player hit her, she was overwhelmed with anxiety about whether she could live up to the standard she had set. As the senior season started, Laura began to feel like an imposter and became so preoccupied with her inadequacies that her game declined. Laura remembers, "I never hit the ball with confidence again. I was so self-conscious that I made simple mistakes and couldn't find a comfortable rhythm with my teammates. Soon I was pulled from the lineup and spent my entire senior season sitting on the bench watching girls with lesser skills playing in my position."

Laura, like many other patients we've worked with, fears success rather than failure. She needs her saboteur to destroy the foundation of that success, because the responsibility seems overwhelming: *What if I let people down? What if I'm not MVP again?* What's scary is trying and failing to reach a goal—to get MVP again, in Laura's case. By not trying or by avoiding the stressful situation, she creates an explanation for her circumstances. The saboteur provides a convenient escape.

Additionally, positive emotions generate more vulnerability than negative ones because they expose us to the potential of rejection, failure, and heartbreak, according to Harvard psychiatrist Dr. George Valiant (Shenk 48). Valiant illustrates his point with the following story. A doctor and well-loved husband retired from his practice of medicine. On his 70th birthday, his wife obtained his patient list and secretly wrote to many of his longstanding patients requesting they write a letter of appreciation to their former physician. She received "100 single-spaced, desperately loving letters—often with pictures attached." His wife put them in a beautiful box covered with Thai silk and gave it to him. Eight years later during a visit from Dr. Valiant, the physician pulled the box of letters down from the shelf and said through tears, "George, I don't know what you'll make of this, but I've never read these." Valiant's conclusion: "It's very hard for most of us to tolerate being loved" (Shenk 48).

Robert was one such man. A survivor of a bitter divorce, he sabotaged one loving relationship after another for more than 15 years until he announced one day in a session, "I think I finally understand what I've been doing to screw up all of these relationships. Once I knew that they had fallen in love with me I found a reason to get rid of them before they had the chance to hurt me. It's strange: All I ever wanted was to be loved, but as soon as someone demonstrates that she's willing to do it, I sabotage the relationship so no one ever hurts me again."

People sabotage themselves in all sorts of ways. Dave, for instance, uses his saboteur to prevent himself from taking the risks necessary to turn his great ideas into great businesses. Dave's friends marvel at his ability to read between the lines with startling accuracy. He envisions things that often come to fruition and seems to understand social and economic trends with unusual clarity. People like to consult Dave about their goals and plans because his approval and blessing inspire confidence and sometimes provide the extra push for people to take action and move forward.

Ironically Dave is a life-long underachiever; he has great talent but has achieved little success. It's not that his ideas lack merit or his plans won't work; it's just that nothing ever comes to fruition because he never takes the risk to invest in his own dreams. His advice and guidance are helpful to other people, but from all indications, Dave will never prosper because he is too afraid of financial ruin and failure. Dave grew up with a stepfather who criticized him mercilessly, liberally using descriptors such "loser" and "failure," and spouting off phrases such as "You'll never amount to anything!" Dave internalized his stepfather's admonitions and contempt, giving birth to his internal saboteur. Of course, no child is a loser, but when Dave made mistakes (which all kids make), he was taught to think of himself that way. Now, his saboteur operates with this self-defeating myth in mind and protects Dave from further failures. Dave is convinced that no matter what he attempts, it won't work. By not applying himself he may avoid failure, but he also contributes to the perception of underachievement. His saboteur makes sure he is locked into a self-fulfilling prophecy: "I know if I try, I'll fail, so I won't try and will merely be an underachiever."

The Saboteur Is Sneaky—Be Aware of How It Operates

It's not just underachievers who are beset by saboteurs. In fact, saboteurs feed on success. This may seem counterintuitive, but keep in mind that nothing buys you immunity from the saboteur within. Doing well in a career or a relationship may make you more fearful of future failure than if you hadn't done well. This doesn't mean you should strive for mediocrity; it simply means you should recognize the devious strategies your saboteur employs to subvert your efforts.

Carrie has a good marriage, two children (a 1-year-old and 3-year-old), and has done well as a business executive. However, she has effectively cut herself off from her friends, her three siblings, and her mother by playing computer solitaire in almost every available spare moment. She even does it at work. Her boss has caught her doing it and warned her to stop. Carrie has played solitaire for years, but it became an obsessive habit when she became a mom and after she received a promotion at work that required more customer contact. It turns out that Carrie's sneaky saboteur is protecting her from an irrational fear of being scorned and reviled during phone calls. As a child, Carrie's family had a party line. Once, when Carrie was 4 years old, she picked up the phone and the person on the line yelled at her loudly and used foul language. It was traumatic for Carrie, and so her saboteur protects her from this happening again by having her spend great amounts of time playing solitaire. In this way, she avoids talking on the phone. When others complain that she never returns calls, Carrie makes the excuse about how busy she is given the new responsibilities of her job and because she's a mother of toddlers. Consciously, Carrie believes this is why she is such a poor phone communicator. In reality, her saboteur encourages her to play solitaire instead of returning calls, in the mistaken belief that this will keep her safe.

Or consider Randy's case. He's succeeded in a number of business ventures, and he projects an aura of leadership and toughness. Nonetheless, his saboteur operates with impunity and with a keen sense of what Randy fears most. As a boy, Randy was gripped by self-doubt. While in middle school, he was the victim of a sexually abusive priest. The incredible shame of being violated by a man led Randy to doubt his own masculinity. This priest also mocked Randy's small penis when he was 11 years old. As a result, he was overcome by feelings of shame, inadequacy, and emasculation. He responded to these feelings by acting tough and angry, looking to fight at a moment's notice. He chose to hang out with a group of guys with whom he could always be the alpha male. With women, however, he often was meek, fearing being laughed at and humiliated. As a result, his saboteur preempted any meaningful relationships with the women Randy met.

Randy tended to succeed in a venture or relationship for a while, only to find some reason to sabotage it later. He had the opportunity to land a prestigious corporate position but feared the public speaking requirements of the job—his saboteur was protecting him from the shame he thought he would feel while "naked" on a stage—and so he turned down a great job. Randy is married to a wonderful woman and has three young kids, but he has had a number of affairs, even though he admits he's not particularly attracted to these other women. It is as if he is hoping these affairs will be discovered and put an end to his successful marriage. Success in any area of his life terrifies Randy, and his internal shame reminds him that he is not deserving of anything but failure. As a result, he has lived life at war with himself—on one hand, trying to overcome the aftermath of the abuse, and on the other, allowing his saboteur to keep him feeling ashamed and emasculated.

Saboteurs thrive during times of internal conflict such as these. They find all sorts of ways to undermine good intentions and booby-trap jobs, relationships, and other meaningful areas of life. Drawing energy from early life traumas, they take advantage of our biggest fears and find a variety of ways to protect us from them. You know the saboteur is talking to you when you hear the same message repeated ad infinitum. For instance, Denise's message is, "You're bad and inadequate." Her internal saboteur makes sure to remind her of stories that prove this message remains true. For instance, Denise often thinks and talks about a 20-year affair she had with a pilot who flew into town once a month to meet her. The pilot was married; she was not. Although the relationship has been over for more than a decade, she believes what she did was wrong, and so she holds onto guilt and the self-deprecatory thoughts ("I'm a bad person"). Without the guilt this oft-remembered story provides she would be free to love again, but she fears that she could not succeed in an intimate relationship. She doesn't believe there is anything inherently lovable about her, nor does she think she has the capacity to make a man happy. Consequently, it is her fear of being intimate that has prompted her to call upon the ready services of the saboteur. The saboteur uses her fear to help her stay away from true intimacy; it reminds her how wrong her affair was and how bad a person she is. If Denise were to allow herself to become seriously involved with someone, she's sure she would ruin things, and she's afraid that the failure of a meaningful relationship would devastate her.

The Ingenious Ways We Self-Sabotage

We are clever in the ways we prevent ourselves from realizing our goals or finding happiness. And we need to be clever, because most of us aren't consciously masochistic and we don't want to admit that we're purposefully messing up our lives. On the surface, we rationalize our self-destructive actions. We provide ourselves with credible excuses for not doing things that could benefit us. In short, we create a plausible cover story for the saboteur.

Let us share an extreme example to demonstrate the lengths we'll go to hide the truth of the saboteur's actions from ourselves. Shirley was suffering from dissociative identity disorder (what used to be called multiple personality disorder). She had engaged a saboteur, but she was not aware of things the saboteur was doing because they were done in the guise of her other personalities. Shirley complained that she couldn't get anything done. The simplest of activities baffled her. Even unloading the dishwasher or helping her daughter prepare for school were suddenly impossible even though she had been doing them successfully for years. She shared her surprise at how she had even gotten to the office for her appointment given how poorly she had been functioning.

In response to questions wondering whether any of her alter-personalities knew what was going on, one of those alters said, "Yeah, I know. We're doing this to her. We're trying to frustrate her because we are afraid of her anger. If she were functioning normally, she might kill her father [for the years of abuse he inflicted upon her]. As long as she can barely put one foot in front of the other, she is not a danger to anyone."

Shirley heard what this alter said and replied, "Okay, I understand. I won't be shooting anybody." Shirley's awareness of her saboteur effectively stopped it from making her dysfunctional. Once she was able to deal with her feelings of anger constructively, she no longer needed to sabotage herself.

We recognize that most of you don't have multiple personality disorder, but we relate this story because it demonstrates how thoroughly a saboteur may control our actions unless we're conscious of it. Think of the internal saboteur as similar to your conscience, only instead of directing you to do what's right, the saboteur keeps you from doing what you fear. By exposing the saboteur—by being aware of your tendencies to act in ways that aren't in your best interest—you take away its power to influence your actions.

Fear isn't the only emotion that causes the tricky saboteur to spring into action. Some people sabotage themselves because they feel resentful and rebellious. Cindy, for instance, is resentful and rebellious because of the way her husband, Jeff, deals with her weight. Though Cindy has tried repeatedly to lose weight, she has failed at diets and other weight loss strategies. Jeff is an avid motorcycle racer and hiker, and he enjoys having Cindy join him in these activities but is worried that her weight gain will prevent her from doing so. As a result, Jeff continuously points out that Cindy has to lose weight. He is not subtle in his negative comments nor is he at all encouraging. Instead, he is persistent, aggressive, and relentless. Cindy calls his approach "the verbal equivalent of a cold sore." She hears questions such as, "Did you go to the gym today? Do you really need to eat that? Do you know how many calories are in one of those?" All of these comments are designed to control Cindy by inducing feelings of guilt.

Cindy resents and rebels against these efforts to control her, but it is virtually impossible for her to lose weight as long as she's rebelling against Jeff's control. Why? Because to lose weight would feel like she was betraying herself and succumbing to Jeff's control. Neither self-betrayal nor submitting to control feels good. So, Cindy unconsciously sabotages her weight loss efforts. She regularly overeats and skips exercise sessions she's promised herself she would attend. On the other hand, when she does manage to lose a pound or two, she finds herself angry and upset as Jeff says, "Okay, 40 more pounds!" or "You see, this isn't so hard, is it? You should have done this years ago!"

So here's the vicious cycle: Cindy feels resentful and controlled, but vows to do better. She drops a few pounds. Jeff comments. Cindy's skin goes prickly. Cindy regains the lost weight plus more. Jeff complains. Cindy chooses therapy over homicide. Ironically, Cindy's rebellion against Jeff culminates in sabotaging her own weight loss, which is not unlike slapping your own face and saying, "There, take that!" Clearly, the internal saboteur appreciates irony. Her rebellion gives it a chance to ensure she keeps the weight on.

Why can't Cindy recognize that she's sabotaging her efforts to lose weight? If you'll recall the Truth from the previous chapter, all behavior has a purpose. Jeff continues to nag Cindy because nagging affords him the illusion of control. To stop nagging would make Jeff feel completely powerless over Cindy's weight (which is a fact he is loathe to acknowledge). He also fears sending the message that he is okay with Cindy's weight; he believes that his silence would cause Cindy to feel okay with being heavy. Therefore, the purpose of Jeff's behavior is to make him feel that he's doing something to correct the problem. Cindy's rebellion gives her a sense of power over Jeff because she resents his control and criticism of her. By sabotaging her own goal of losing weight, she also avoids dealing with other difficult issues, including any unhappiness in her relationship with Jeff and any painful, unresolved issues from her childhood. As we've noted, avoiding discomfort is a very human tendency. Avoidance provides immediate relief. Cindy avoids her difficulties, eats for comfort, and continues to maintain her weight, much to Jeff's and her own disgust.

Rebellion and resentment cause our saboteur to act against our own self-interest. Mike, a 30-year-old opiate abuser, resents his mother's efforts to control his rehab so much that he is tempted to return to substance abuse to show her who is boss. Angie, an 18-year-old woman, resents her father because of his "old-world Italian control." He insists that she go to college; she decides she'll show him and drops out of high school. Given that the saboteur operates under cover of resentment, rebellion, and fear, how can we get it under control? The best approach is to understand and work with the saboteur rather than against it. In this way, you can take advantage of the energy it brings to the party.

Six Steps to Keep Your Saboteur Under Control

The following actions can help you outfox your internal saboteur without trying to assassinate him. Keep in mind that your saboteur is trying to protect you, and that he brings ingenuity and motivation to his efforts. You want to retain these positives and direct them at worthwhile goals. This six-step process will be useful in that regard.

1. Embrace

The saboteur is like a big brother who defends us on the playground from the lunch-stealing bully. It acts as our friend and protector. As such, it is not something we want to eliminate entirely. The impulse to protect ourselves from things we fear is a good one, and part of our survival instinct. Somehow, though, our internal saboteur becomes separated from who we are and what we really need. Therefore, try to integrate the saboteur back into who you are at your core. Embrace the self-protective side of the saboteur, but at the same time, be aware which fears are illusory and which are real. Your saboteur takes your lead from you, and so you need to confide in it what really matters in your life. By embracing the saboteur, you're recognizing your tendencies to act in ways that aren't in your best interest. This consciousness will help you protect yourself from the saboteur's misguided attempts to protect you.

2. Address

Identify what the saboteur is fighting. What is your fear, and what does this fear say about you? If you're afraid of failure, try to understand where that fear came from and what that fear says about you. Determine if you're like Randy, and your saboteur is protecting you based on a traumatic incident when you were a child. Rethink who you are and what you're capable of becoming. Don't accept your self-defeating behaviors. Recognize that you're scared, resentful, or rebellious, and that you must figure out exactly what it is you're scared of, resentful about or rebelling against. When you address these issues, you diminish the power of the saboteur.

3. Adapt

You can't continue to operate the same way you always have. Once you address why and how the saboteur acts, you need to be realistic with yourself about what you must do differently. Be realistic, even if it hurts. For instance, if your fear of intimacy causes your saboteur to keep you from pursuing relationships, determine why you fear intimacy. Is it the belief that you don't know how to be intimate? Based on what you discover, you must learn and adapt. Avoidance only leads to greater fear. Also, recognize that as you adapt and try new behaviors, you may fail. For instance, you fear intimacy, but you manage to find someone whom you really like and then she rejects you. Though it might not feel like it at the time, failure is important. If we're not failing, we're not growing. Reflect upon the failure and learn from it, because that's the source of wisdom.

There was a Michael Jordan commercial in which he admitted that he missed more than 9,000 shots in his career. Of these, 27 were in the final seconds of a game that his team ultimately lost. Considered one of the greatest winners in the history of sports, Michael admitted that his success came from failing repeatedly and striving to overcome his failures. He adapted and became even better than he already was.

4. Plan

Create a plan based on the previous three steps in such as way that you both embrace and release fear. If your plan represents only token change, then it probably won't make you fearful—or do you any good. Susan Jeffers wrote a book titled, *Feel the Fear and Do It Anyway*. This is your planning guideline. Fear, like any other human emotion, is brought about by perception. If you perceive something to be dangerous and/or threatening, feel that feeling, release it, and then think differently about what you're so afraid of. Make sure your plan also keeps you alert for catastrophic thinking—the idea that things are awful, terrible, or headed for a potential catastrophe. Your saboteur relishes this type of thinking, as it causes a lot of fear and makes you willing to act against your best interests to avoid that fear. Your plan should substitute what-is-the-worst-that-could-happen questioning for the catastrophic thinking.

5. Act

A plan that gathers dust is no plan at all. Make a conscious effort to implement your plan. When you do, be sure to include your saboteur in your implementation effort. Don't ignore its existence. Instead, when you start trying new behaviors, ask your saboteur to reframe its role. For instance, Steve was a patent attorney filled with self-doubt. In the past, his saboteur wouldn't let him try anything new or take any risks, especially professionally. As part of the plan, Steve asked his saboteur to remain his protector, but to do so differently. Instead of telling him that he was a failure and could not achieve because he was not smart enough, he would protect him by reinforcing his positive self-image before, during, and after a risk-taking endeavor. Steve also asked his saboteur to avoid looking at his new behaviors in black-and-white terms. In other words, Steve knew that when he moved out and tried new things, he would sometimes fail. He requested that his saboteur speak to him about it without seeing a failure as a stupid mistake; rather, that he recognize that it was a necessary learning step toward ultimate success. As a result, when Steve began acting on his plan, he found that the saboteur felt much more like a supportive friend than an internal tormentor. He incorporated the passion, energy, and self-protective nature of the saboteur rather than continue to run from it or battle it directly.

6. Thrive

The last step is resolving to move forward in a positive direction, even if things go awry. This positive attitude in the face of setbacks keeps the saboteur from doing any damage. Too often, people embark on a new life plan, suffer a setback, and globalize the negative results. You may fail your math test, but that doesn't make you a failure. You may not have studied hard enough or the test may have been a tough one. A positive but realistic outlook thwarts the saboteur. As long as you recognize that you're capable, intelligent, and courageous enough to take a risk, and resilient enough to start over if things don't go well, your saboteur won't cause you to act in self-destructive ways.

Use coping statements in order to thrive. Statements such as "I can stand it if we lose this game" or "it is not the end of the world if our bid is not accepted by the company" and "I am lovable and deserving of love regardless of whether the person I desire chooses to love me" work well. Remember, the most important aspect of any situation is what you tell yourself about it. Your nervous system will respond only to your beliefs and conclusions, not the objective reality of the situation.

All six steps should be used when you're in situations in which you're most inclined to sabotage yourself. You know what those situations are, whether they involve work, romantic relationships, or family. Although it may feel awkward at first to think about these six steps and put them into practice, they'll soon become second nature. As you discover that they stop you from shooting yourself in the foot when you try something new or risky, then you'll be that much more motivated to make them part of your daily routine.

Now let's try some exercises that will help you deal with your internal saboteur in positive ways.

Exercises

Exercise 1—Identify the Saboteur's M.O. (Modus Operandi)

The following questions are designed to help you determine how your saboteur operates. As you now know, this identification process is important, because the more you know about it, the better you'll be able to manage it. After each question, we've included some possible responses to facilitate identification. Check any that apply to you.

1. What does your saboteur keep you from achieving?
    - ❑ Reaching job goals
    - ❑ Satisfying romantic relationships
    - ❑ Maintaining or creating new friendships
    - ❑ Spending time productively
    - ❑ Relaxing/spending time on a hobby
    - ❑ Attaining financial security
    - ❑ Other _____

2. When does your saboteur appear?

   ❏ When I'm under a great deal of stress.

   ❏ When I'm on the cusp of achieving an objective in my life.

   ❏ When I'm starting to feel good about myself.

   ❏ When I'm angry about something.

   ❏ Other _____

3. What do you fear and what does this fear say about you?

   ❏ Having a serious relationship; it says I'm afraid of being destroyed if the relationship fails.

   ❏ Being successful in my career; it says I'm afraid of finding my dream job and then blowing it.

   ❏ Being responsible for others—a spouse, kids, employees; it says that I'm afraid that I won't live up to this responsibility.

   ❏ Other _____

4. What might you be apprehensive about if the saboteur were not present to protect you?

   ❏ Moving in with my significant other.

   ❏ Being promoted.

   ❏ Relocating to the place I've always dreamed about.

   ❏ Taking on a leadership role.

   ❏ Losing weight and keeping it off.

   ❏ Other _____

5. Where did this apprehension originate?

   ❏ Something my parent(s) did or said when I was a child.

   ❏ A traumatic childhood experience unrelated to my family.

   ❏ A failed adult relationship.

   ❏ A catastrophic work experience.

   ❏ Other _____

Exercise 2—What's the Worst That Can Happen?

The negative voice of the saboteur comes from your fear of what might happen. You've catastrophized what is merely uncomfortable or unpleasant. This exercise is designed to help you confront the worst that can happen and recognize that it's not as horrible as you think.

1. Given what you fear most, describe the worst possible outcomes you can imagine based on this fear:

   _____

   _____

   _____

2. Has this worst possible outcome ever taken place? Describe what has happened because of your fear. How far removed is it from your worst possible outcome?

   _____

   _____

   _____

3. Now imagine for a moment that your worst possible outcome comes to pass. Write three possible responses to it you might have that could help you minimize the damage. Then describe three actions you might take that might help you rebound from this negative situation:

   _____

   _____

   _____

   _____

Exercise 3—The Six Steps

With the previous exercises in mind, you're now ready to put the six steps discussed in the chapter into action. By now you know your saboteur well and are aware that it's protecting you from something that isn't as awful as you may have feared. With this knowledge as your foundation, take the following steps:

1. Embrace: Write a statement acknowledging what the saboteur tries to do to keep you safe. Include in the statement the pattern of protection that keeps recurring. Make sure your statement reflects your recognition that the saboteur is acting in your best interest; seek understanding of its motives rather than trying to destroy it.

_____

_____

_____

2. Address: Address the fear, resentment, and rebellion that cause the saboteur to act on your behalf, and create a statement of what you would prefer that it help you do—specifically, how this internal bodyguard might help you act, think, or feel differently.

_____

_____

_____

3. Adapt: What lessons can you learn from your saboteur that will enable you to change and be willing to risk failure? Specify at least two ways you hope to change your behaviors.

_____

_____

_____

4. Plan: Create a plan for dealing with your saboteur. This plan should be a simple series of actions designed to deal effectively with the saboteur when it attempts to protect you from what you fear most. What will you do (and think and feel) differently when x occurs? Plan alternative ways of responding to common situations to which you're vulnerable.

    _____

    _____

    _____

5. Act: Make a commitment to act at a specific time, place, and situation. In the following space, affirm your willingness to act in a different way the next time your saboteur surfaces. Create an affirmation such as, "The next time I meet someone I like and I find myself thinking about cutting off contact, I promise to make a date for us to do something the next weekend."

    _____

    _____

    _____

    _____

6. Thrive: Reinforce the positive outcome of acting in a more conscious, fearless way by stating the benefits you'll reap. List at least three benefits that will be yours if you don't sabotage yourself.

    _____

    _____

    _____

Chapter 5

All Behavior Requires Permission, So We Must Learn What We're Permitting Ourselves to Do

Be the master of your will and the slave of your conscience.

—Anonymous

Human behavior is constantly amazing—and perplexing. A young man home from college walks into his sleeping sister's bedroom and touches her inappropriately. She awakens to the violation and then tells her parents, who are outraged. How could he do such a thing? It is not unusual for a young man to be driven by sexual feelings, nor is it odd for a male to want to touch the body of a female. The horror in this situation comes from the young man's sexual exploitation of a sleeping, non-consenting person who is his sister. These three factors make his behavior entirely unacceptable, if not illegal. How does someone bring himself to make such a decision? How did this young man give himself permission to act so outrageously?

This fifth Truth—all human behavior requires permission—gives you unprecedented control over how you behave in different situations. You may think you're a pawn in other people's games or that you respond by unthinking reflex; but, in fact, you control the picture. The Truth is that you're the one who gives yourself permission to act in certain ways. I (Chris) was first introduced to this concept while taking a driver's course after I had been caught speeding. The instructor commented that we speed because we give ourselves permission to exceed the speed limit. He then presented a coherent argument why it is in our best interest to obey the speed limit and other traffic laws, but his point about permission resonated with me. I speed because I have permission from myself to go faster than the law allows! Further, I need my own permission to yell at another human being, rob a convenience store at gunpoint, cheat on my spouse, or eat an entire bag of candy. *But wait*, you say, *I didn't give myself permission to eat that bag of candy; I just saw it, got hungry, and ate it.* It was pure reaction, and there was no permission involved. Or, perhaps you simply were not aware of when and how you gave yourself permission.

Behavior Doesn't Just Happen

Try this experiment. Think back to when you first learned the difference between good and bad, right and wrong. Is stealing good or bad? Is saying something disrespectful to an adult acceptable? Is it okay to lie? Most people say these lessons are internalized between the ages of 3 and 8. Now consider when you began to live by that standard of good versus bad or right versus wrong. If you're like most people, you may have started trying to apply this standard early in life, but still find yourself struggling with this issue. You're not sure if you should take a great job with a company responsible for environmental pollution. You don't want to lie and mislead your girlfriend that you will eventually get married, but you fear that if you are completely honest with her, she'll break up with you. You don't have hard-and-fast rules that you follow in all circumstances that govern your behavior. You may be honest in one instance but not so honest in the next. How you act depends on the circumstance.

When you act dishonestly or in a way that is mean-spirited or self-destructive, you're doing so with malice aforethought. In other words, you have a choice, and you've chosen to give yourself permission to act that way. A man reported that his wife sometimes hits him when she is very angry. He said that his previous therapist asked him why his wife hit him. He would then try to explain the entire argument to the best of his ability, including her rationale for hitting him. In fact, the reason his wife hits him is very simple—she has given herself permission to hit him when she is angry. Most people never lift a hand against their spouses when they are angry with them. Likewise, they don't hit their children, even though they may spank them for misbehaving.

Most men learn early on that it is unmanly to hit a girl. They lack permission to strike a female under any circumstance. Soon, these men have internalized this message, and for this reason, they never do it. They do not grant themselves permission to act that way, and without permission, they can't act.

You can also look at this issue from another angle. Think of those who do abuse their spouses. They have granted themselves permission to hit their wife or husband. They are violent people. Yet why don't they also hit their boss at work, whom they clearly dislike? Why don't they get into physical confrontations with friends during arguments? Because they have only granted themselves permission for violent behavior with their spouse.

When we grant ourselves permission to do something we previously considered unacceptable, problem behaviors begin. Marijuana is called the gateway drug because many people start abusing other, harder drugs once they've used it. When they permit themselves to use marijuana, a psychological boundary line is crossed; there is now permission to use other illegal drugs. It has become acceptable to have mind-altering experiences through drugs, and subsequently it's not a great leap from marijuana to other mind-altering substances. The great leap is from using no drugs at all to smoking marijuana, as this requires permission from the self to engage in an illegal act. Consider the following research from the National Household Survey on Drug Abuse (1993). The report indicates that once someone makes a choice to participate in risky behaviors such as using drugs, the potential to engage in other such behaviors increases significantly. The use of one drug directly correlates to the use of other drugs. If a child smokes or drinks alcohol, he or she is 65 times more likely to use marijuana than a child who never smokes or drinks. If a child smokes marijuana even once in his or her lifetime, he/she is 104 times more likely to use cocaine than a child who never used marijuana.

Drug abuse is not the only problem behavior that requires permission from self. Infidelity, contrary to popular belief, does not just happen between two unsuspecting people. They are neither victims of love and lust, nor are they random individuals who passively "fall in love." The truth is, having an affair requires a series of decisions wherein two individuals grant themselves permission to engage in conversation and behaviors that promote infidelity. For example, we need permission to talk about how our current relationship is making us unhappy, how the sex is unsatisfying, and how we dream about a more fulfilling relationship. Likewise, we must give ourselves permission to send clandestine e-mails, obtain secret cell phones, and meet for private lunches or weekends. An affair is neither an accident nor a single decision, but rather a series of sanctioned thoughts and behaviors that comprise the relationship. People who have affairs are not necessarily in worse relationships than people who don't; they simply have given themselves permission to think and behave in ways that allow infidelity to occur.

As impulsive as violent behavior may appear to be, it is born out of self-granted permission. This permission is often deeply rooted in childhood lessons taught by your father—for instance, "A man rules the roost by whatever means necessary." Even though the origin of the permission may be in the distant past, you must reapply for permission to exercise this behavior in the present. Domestic violence prevention programs across the country teach abusers to be mindful of their thinking, especially thoughts that encourage violent behavior such as "If she opens her fat mouth one more time, I'll shut it for her," or "I need to show her that she can't treat me disrespectfully," or "I don't have to tolerate her crap." Such thinking presupposes permission to abuse someone if certain conditions arise. As suggested earlier, this same abusive spouse would not hit his boss under any circumstance, because there is no permission to do so.

Children are often rude and disrespectful to their parents. These same children wouldn't dream of disrespecting teachers, neighbors, clergy, or police officers in the same way. Why the discrepancy? They have permission from themselves and their parents to behave that way. All behavior requires permission. Permission is necessary to sneak into a movie or write a movie, follow or break a diet, insult or compliment a stranger, buy or sell a dream house.

Just as we give ourselves permission for all that we do, we also give others permission to treat us in certain ways. Dr. Phil McGraw, the well-known television psychologist, asserts that we actually teach people how to treat us. That is, when we don't object or remove ourselves from abusive language, physical aggression, or persistent threats, we are, in fact, giving someone permission to treat us in an unacceptable manner. We may permit others to tease us mercilessly, use us financially, disrespect us publicly, or even cheat on us sexually, merely by the way we respond to those behaviors. Some people make it very clear early in relationships that such behavior will not be tolerated, thereby setting psychologically healthy boundaries (a Truth that will be discussed in Chapter 7).

We also give others permission to love us. Conversely, some of us withhold this permission because we don't love or respect ourselves, preventing others from being close to us emotionally, physically, or sexually. We fear that we are not worthy, that if we allow others to get close, they'll figure out that we're not lovable and reject us. Contrary to the romantic Hollywood stereotype, we don't simply fall in love when the right person comes along; we first need to grant ourselves permission to love and be loved.

Permission to Change

Just as our behavior requires permission, so, too, does changing behavior. If we don't grant ourselves permission to move away from existing counterproductive behavior, we'll keep falling back into these routines no matter how negative their outcomes might be. An oft-quoted Bible story, taken from John 8:1–8, makes this point well. An adulteress is about to be stoned by an angry crowd. Jesus approaches the mob and suggests that whoever is without sin should cast the first stone, whereupon everyone drops their stones and walks away. Jesus then asks the adulteress, "Where are your accusers?" He continues, "Neither do I accuse you. Go and sin no more." Clergy teach this story as a cautionary tale to pound home the message that "judge not, lest ye be judged." What is relevant for our purposes, however, is the instruction Jesus gives the adulteress: "Go and sin no more." Jesus clearly believes that she can cease and desist from her behavior; he is telling her to stop giving herself permission to sin. The implication is that she has the capacity to retract the self-granted permission to conduct extramarital relationships and to think differently about matters of fidelity and relationships. Clearly, Jesus was aware that all changes in behavior begin with the decision to retract permission and think differently.

For example, the Alcoholics Anonymous program teaches the recovering alcoholic to think differently about alcohol. The first of the program's 12 steps asserts, "I am powerless over alcohol, and my life has become unmanageable." They now recognize alcohol as something that has the power to control and destroy their life, so they remove permission to use alcohol or even to think of alcohol as being an answer to temporary problems or an outlet for recreational pursuits. Recovering alcoholics believe that one drink will become an endless number of drinks, making even a sip unacceptable. To resume drinking after a period of abstinence requires permission from self—permission that the recovering alcoholic learns to withhold. This principle is illustrated in the movie, *The House of Sand and Fog*, in which the female lead, played by Jennifer Connelly, dates a police officer who drinks and encourages her to do so as well. The audience sees her painfully looking at the bottle and wondering if she should permit herself to give in and imbibe for the first time in many months. Her turmoil culminates in a "what the hell" decision. She takes the drink, which is the beginning of a series of disasters in her life.

Retracting permission is necessary for anyone who wants to change any type of behavior, including habitual lying, late-night snacking, or watching pornography. Only a decision to remove permission to do any of these things and a necessary plan to accomplish that goal will be effective. The half-hearted "let's see how it goes" mentality generally is ineffective, even for people with the best of intentions. The best predictor of future behavior is past behavior, so unless you make a firm commitment to remove permission and make a plan to do something else, you are likely to continue doing what you have always done.

How to Change Behavior: Permit Yourself to Take Six Steps

Initially, it may seem a simple matter of resolving not to give yourself permission for routine counterproductive behaviors, but if you've ever tried to quit an addiction—smoking, drinking, drugs—you know how difficult it can be to stop these behaviors. Even less serious behaviors, such as an inability to commit to a relationship or the tendency to sabotage your career, can be extraordinarily difficult to give up. For this reason, it helps to have a process by which you formally grant yourself permission to change how you act. Let's examine each of the six steps in this process.

Step 1: Be aware that a particular behavior is a problem. The adulterous woman was aware of her problem when the mob clutched the stones in their hands ready to fire. Better to be aware of the need for change *before* the stoning than when it's about to happen. You don't want to be caught with your third DUI or find yourself losing someone who might have been Mr. or Ms. Right because you waited too long to gain awareness of your problem. Therefore, focus on what's going wrong in your life. Talk to the people closest to you—friends, family, trusted work colleagues—and ask them what they've observed. The odds are they'll be able to identify your behavioral problems, even if you can't. By improving your awareness of what's wrong, you gain insight into the problem. This insight helps you identify the behavior that needs to be changed and paves the way for you to give yourself permission to change it.

Step 2: Decide to change. Here is where you revoke permission to engage in negative behaviors. You tell yourself you are no longer allowed to eat whatever you want, whenever you want. You forbid yourself to lapse into a catatonic state every weekend, never going out and meeting other people. You insist to yourself that you will no longer look for and accept low-paying jobs that fail to challenge you. Understand that when you revoke permission, you have to mean it. You can't say that you'll see how it goes before committing to the revocation of permission. You can't qualify the revocation; it must be unequivocal.

Step 3: Establish a goal. Abstaining from alcohol, balancing your budget, and completing a master's degree are excellent goals because they are specific and measurable. These are more likely to lead to success than more general goals such as "I hope to drink less" or "I want a better education." Goals need to be objective, attainable, measurable, and quantifiable. Your goal helps you lay the groundwork for new behaviors that are permissible, providing guidance as you move forward.

Step 4: Develop a specific plan to attain the goal. Losing a considerable amount of weight, for instance, is possible but usually requires a definite plan as to how to accomplish it. Walking two miles every morning and following a 1,500-calorie regimen is a more specific plan than "I'm going to exercise more and eat less." Breaking the plan into increments—small, attainable tasks—facilitates achieving the goal. Maybe you start out walking half a mile every morning, then move to one mile after a week, and so on. Remember, when you deny yourself permission to do one thing and grant permission to do a new thing, you may feel a bit uncomfortable initially. Specifically planned tasks diminish the discomfort.

Step 5: Work the plan. A plan is only as effective as your ability to execute it. Many people fall off the wagon when attempting to change behaviors. Human nature almost guarantees unplanned deviations from the original itinerary. Nonetheless, studies tell us that the more you persevere toward achieving a goal, the better your chance of attaining it. To wit, people who repeatedly attempt to quit smoking cigarettes have a greater chance of finally quitting. One study of battered spouses suggested that a person has to leave home an average of four times before he or she can finally leave the relationship permanently. To persevere, repeat to yourself what you no longer are permitting yourself to do. This will help reinforce the lessons learned from the past, and provide an incentive to stay with the plan.

Step 6: Alter the routine. A number of recovery programs offer a colloquial definition of insanity: doing the same thing over and over again and expecting different results. My favorite example of this form of insanity comes from watching couples in marital counseling. The couple follows the same predictable dance steps in all of their fights: attack, defend, counterattack, and withdraw; repeat as necessary; and wonder why they can't seem to improve their relationship. The couple may break up, resume contact, get back together, and try more sincerely than ever before. Unfortunately, they fall back into old patterns and the relationship fails. Change can only take place when the couple understands the dance and the predictable outcome.

Know your destructive routines. Be aware of the insidious patterns that draw you in. Remind yourself regularly that you no longer have permission to fall into these routines and patterns. Give yourself permission to embrace behaviors that disrupt the routine. In this way, you can create new, healthier patterns.

Permission to Seek Challenges

Here is an example from my practice of a child's giving himself permission to hurt others and later retracting that permission. Two bullies roughed up one of my teenage clients at his high school. Despite his reporting the abuse to the proper authorities, nothing was done. Only after another kicking and choking scene was caught on the school's security camera did the authorities get involved. In fact, the police resource officer pressed charges against the bullies. In court, one of the bullies failed to appear; the other wrote a long apology letter to my client that explained why and how he had become a bully. Note the permission-giving sequence in his letter:

> Dear Edward:
>
> I'm really sorry that I kept hitting you and picking on you at school. I know it's no excuse, but I want you to know that I was bullied by Greg too. When I was in 6th grade, he used to hit me and grind his knuckles into my head. He even took a new watch I got for my birthday and threatened to kill me if I told anyone. One day he told me he'd stop picking on me if I agreed to "accidently" knock over the art project of this kid he hated and called "Goody Two Shoes." I knew it was wrong, but I decided to do it anyway so Greg would leave me alone. When I saw the boy cry after his art project was destroyed, I felt bad but I tried not to care. Greg was so excited. It's kind of dumb but I wanted Greg to like me so I decided not to care about anyone else's feelings. It's weird but the more I picked on other kids the more Greg wanted to hang out with me. And another thing happened. I stopped feeling so bad when I hurt people.

Even you. Except now I feel really bad, Edward, because I know I really hurt you and I remember how scared I was when Greg used to pick on me. All I can say is I'm really, really sorry, Edward, and I'll never do anything like this to anyone again.

Sincerely, Justin

Clearly, we can determine that what prompted Justin to grant himself permission to behave as a bully was his fear of Greg and a desire for his approval. Interestingly, it was also Justin's fear—this time, of consequences and guilt—that led him to retract his permission to continue on the path of being the school thug. As long as he continues to retract that permission, he will never play the bully again.

Following are exercises to help you apply Truth # 5 to your life.

Exercises

Exercise 1—What Do I Do Over and Over Again?

Many people struggle to identify their problem behaviors—the counterproductive routines and negative patterns, which Freud called *repetition compulsion*. Though you probably think you know what your compulsively repeated behaviors are, this is not necessarily so. That's because you've rationalized or denied them, which prevents you from being aware of what they are. This exercise is designed to foster this awareness.

The following list includes some common repeated behavioral problems. Make a check next to any that apply to you:

❑ Sabotaging relationships before they become serious.

❑ Doing everything possible to limit your success.

❑ Becoming hostile and angry under stress.

❑ Demeaning those who mean the most to you.

❑ Committing obvious, detrimental mistakes at work.

❑ Spending more money than you have.

❑ Engaging in the same knock-down, drag-out arguments with those who love you most.

❑ Worrying constantly about what might happen.

❑ Paying little or no attention (or too much attention) to your appearance.

❑ Drinking or gambling to excess.

❑ Rebelling against anyone in authority.

❑ Being able to function effectively in the presence of authority figures.

❑ Disordered eating.

❑ Spending all your time and energy on work and ignoring other aspects of your life.

(If none of these repeated problem behaviors apply to you, see if you can use them to create your own list.)

Exercise 2—Why Do I Do It?

The goal of this exercise is to help you understand why you give yourself permission to engage in your repeated negative behaviors. We've listed six strategies people use when they permit themselves to act counterproductively. See which strategy applies to you and recognize that it's deceptive and that you're endorsing a permission that is bad for you. Then describe how you use this strategy in your life.

1. Justification: You make a judgment that makes sense to you so you can engage in an unhealthy behavior. "It's her fault I hit her because she made me so angry." What's your justification?

_____

_____

_____

2. Minimization: You admit to choosing an unhealthy behavior but assert that it is not significant or important. "Yeah, I went off my diet and ate three desserts, but it's no big deal." How do you minimize your actions?

_____

_____

_____

_____

3. Rationalization: You create excuses or alibis for your behavior. "Officer, I was speeding because I am late," or "My dog ate my homework." What do you rationalize?

_____

_____

_____

_____

4. Intellectualization: You allow yourself to engage in unhealthy behaviors by removing your emotions from the decision-making process. "What do you mean, I have a problem with pot? It's better to have a high society than a drunken society," or "Come on, everybody cheats on their taxes." How do you intellectualize your negative choices?

_____

_____

_____

5. Denial: You claim you did not engage in a particular behavior when you did. "I did not have inappropriate sexual relations with that woman." What behaviors do you deny?

    _____

    _____

    _____

    _____

6. Externalization: You place the blame on someone else. "It's not my responsibility," or "You should have reminded me." Whom do you blame for your unhealthy choices?

    _____

    _____

    _____

    _____

Chapter 6

Emotional Energy Is Finite and Needs to Be Invested, Rather Than Wasted on Wishing, Worrying, and Whining

That which dominates our imagination and thoughts will determine our lives and character.

—Ralph Waldo Emerson

Sports Illustrated runs an occasional feature titled "Where Are They Now?" to keep readers informed about the activities of retired star athletes who have stepped out of the spotlight. In the July 12–19, 2004 issue, the magazine also included a feature titled "No Longer Busts." These stories covered athletes who were highly touted in their college careers and were expected to be superstars but never lived up to the hype, and who were sometimes shamed and ridiculed because of their failures. The athletes profiled are "no longer busts" because they found a way to handle their failures and move on to rewarding careers in other fields. What does all this have to do with this chapter's Truth? It's not that they found success in another area of life; rather, they developed a healthy perspective on perceived failure. Rather than wasting energy bemoaning and lamenting the past, they learned from their experiences, which led them to successful and meaningful endeavors apart from sports.

Many people spend their lives living in regret and resentment about things that did not turn out the way they had hoped and planned. What people fail to recognize is that their expression of resentment wastes precious personal energy. The Truth is we need to conserve this energy and invest it in activities and goals that matter. This Truth may seem self-evident, but people often act as if their energy is unlimited and that it doesn't matter if they fritter it away on regrets or complaints. To help you recognize all the ways in which you may be wasting your personal energy, let's look a bit deeper at how this waste occurs.

Conserving Precious Resources

Think about how much time you spend rationalizing, complaining, and replaying past events. More specifically, think of one particular recent example of rationalization. For instance:

- ▶ "My boss doesn't respect me; that's why I haven't been promoted."

- ▶ "The police officer needed to satisfy his quota; that's why I was pulled over for speeding."

- ▶ "He didn't ask me out because he's so busy with his work."

These rationalizations reflect a personal choice to focus on factors that are external to us and beyond our control. What particular justification have you relied on recently that involves something beyond your control? The odds are a rationalization immediately popped into your mind. Most of us use a lot of energy to create these justifications in our heads. They require a lot of mulling and the creation of illogical conclusions. We also tend to dwell on our rationalizations, spending a lot of time and emotional energy examining them as a child would a new toy. If you do this too often—if you spend a significant part of your day rationalizing, complaining, or dwelling on the past—it suggests a life lacking fulfillment. You may not only be unproductive in your work, but you may also be frustrated because you're not achieving your personal dreams. This happens because you are investing your energy in the wrong place.

If you think about your available energy as a finite mathematical construct, the value of investing it wisely becomes clearer. Human beings, regardless of race, color, creed, or socioeconomic status, have 24 hours a day to live. They also have a limited amount of emotional energy to expend in that 24-hour period. Imagine that we could quantify emotional energy by asserting that each of us has 100 units of energy to spend in the course of a day in any way we choose. We are free to think whatever thoughts and to engage in whatever behaviors strike our fancy. The energy does not carry over to tomorrow; the 100 units must be used today or be lost.

For instance, let's say you wake up in the morning and whine about your boss. That uses up 20 units of energy. Then, on your train ride into work, you obsess about a relationship that didn't work out, replaying how this person broke up with you and wishing it had gone differently. There goes another 15 units. When you arrive at work and turn on your computer, you learn that the stock market plummeted and your industry has been especially hard hit. There goes another 15 units of energy, spent worrying that you might not have a job for long.

Before lunch, you have spent half of your daily supply of energy units. You may go through the motions at work, but you're not going to be particularly productive or derive much satisfaction from what you do. You'll have trouble concentrating. You may have a date later in the evening, but you're not going to be good company. In essence, you squandered a significant amount of your energy units on unproductive thinking. Who knows? Perhaps if you had saved a substantial portion of those energy units, you might have had a breakthrough idea that won you a promotion or made a great impression with a date you truly cared about. The harm done by squandering this energy isn't just that it's wasted, but that it's not available for activities that matter. Think of all the opportunities missed and problems not solved because you were enervated or distracted before noon—not just for one day, but for many days out of your life! In therapy, we sometimes refer to the adage that "some people complain that rose bushes have thorns, while other people rejoice that thorn bushes have roses." Focusing on the positive conserves your energy for things that matter.

Now consider the athletes we referred to earlier, the ones who made comebacks from being busts. They could have used their energy to harp on what might have been, but somewhere along the way, they chose not to live in frustration and regret. Instead, they invested their energy wisely in activities that promoted their lives and the lives of their families and their communities. Athletes are encouraged to have short-term memories, and we would encourage you to do the same, at least in terms of negative events. If you focus on the past you are not focusing on the one reality, which is the present.

You can make the choice to live in the moment. It's a question of making yourself aware of how you spend your energy rather than wasting it unconsciously. To create this awareness, you need to learn the three ways that people waste their emotional energy: 1) wishing the past was different, 2) worrying about the future, and 3) whining about the uncontrollable aspects of life.

Wishing the Past Was Different

Don is a 52-year-old gentleman who came to therapy to work on several issues, relationships being the most pressing. He had had remarkably few encounters with the opposite sex in his five decades. Consequently, he had spent much of his time questioning, regretting, and wondering about the few dates he'd had. Every day he wondered what might have been if one of the women he liked had not moved away. He just as regularly regretted not having asked a woman out on a date when he had the opportunity. He put so much time and energy into the "what ifs" that he failed to focus on relationships in the present. We're not suggesting you should never think about or learn from the past. What this Truth really suggests is that you should learn from the past so you can invest your energy on the present and plan to do things differently.

Consider that people who constantly wish upon the past are like people who only listen to a radio's oldie station. Although it's fun to relive past memories and events, we experience no new music while listening to this station. Musically, we are stuck in another era and stunted in our development of music appreciation. Imagine if life is lived so that we do not move forward because our emotional energy is devoted primarily to something that happened long ago—a broken marriage, a failed business, or a betrayal by a trusted friend or lover. Perhaps self-pity affords us some satisfaction as we replay the perceived violations and negative events from our past, but it prevents us from getting on with our lives.

Don would have done well to "live and learn" from his past mistakes. He could have acknowledged his unhelpful or unhealthy behaviors and made a plan to implement different behaviors. He could have used his time and energy to meet appropriate women in his life now, rather than repeatedly dredging up and dissecting his few encounters years ago. It is a human tendency to return to unfinished incidences or experiences, and the reliving of them can be enervating. Making peace with the unfinished past facilitates living in the present. As the saying goes, "he who is blind to the past, is doomed to relive it."

Phil was a fascinating man in his mid-50s, a well-dressed professional with a refined vocabulary and a no-nonsense attitude. He was also highly accomplished with two master's degrees, several businesses, and a run for Congress under his belt. Phil had a room devoted to the accomplishments in his life. The walls of the room were covered with numerous plaques that boasted of his achievements in the academic, political, and business worlds. When he began to run out of space on the walls in this room, he created another room in the house that he could use for displaying plaques. When I asked Phil what his plaque room was really about, he shook his head and said, "I'm not sure." After thinking about it for a while, he said, "I suppose what I really want is a visit from my father. I'd like him to walk into the room, look up at all the plaques and say to me, 'Son, I'm proud of you.'"

It turned out that Phil was devoting the bulk of his time and emotional and physical energy to one thing—gaining the approval of his father. Ironically, Phil recalled that his father was incapable of saying approving words because his own life was marked by a great deal of personal pain and trauma, not to mention alcoholism. He never communicated what he felt for Phil positively, but instead his words came out in the form of criticism and denigration. Regardless of his extraordinary accomplishments, Phil could not get something from his father that his father was incapable of giving. Yet he persisted in spending his daily allotment of emotional energy on a past that couldn't be changed. Although Phil achieved a lot despite this restraint, he placed an artificial ceiling on his achievements because he was so focused on the past. More to the point, Phil couldn't fully enjoy his achievements because of his backward-looking gaze.

Worrying About the Future

In this volatile, unpredictable age, people worry more about the future than they did during times of economic stability and prosperity. They expend huge amounts of energy creating "what-if" possibilities. They agonize over worst-case scenarios. They spend countless hours fretting and fuming over everything from economic to interpersonal disasters. Think about whether you have invested energy in worrying about the following future negative events:

What will happen to your job if…

- ▶ Your boss decides to retire or is fired?
- ▶ Your industry or the economy suffers a downturn?
- ▶ A new technology emerges that makes your skills obsolete?

These are all reasonable questions, but obsessing about them when there's nothing you can do to prevent them is nonsensical. Yet people read an article or see a news report and it triggers a string of what-ifs about their job or industry. It gives them insomnia, headaches, and upset stomachs, but no matter how hard they worry, it doesn't give them any relief.

What will happen to your money if…

- ▶ Your neighborhood starts going downhill?
- ▶ We have a real depression instead of a serious recession?
- ▶ You are no longer able to retire when you planned (because of unexpected healthcare costs, for example)?

Again, we are at the mercy of economic forces beyond our control, and focusing our time and attention on what might happen isn't going to alter those forces one bit. You can do as many spread sheets as you want and do as much research as possible, but you can't prepare for every economic contingency (though you certainly can worry about it incessantly).

What will happen to your significant other if…

- ▶ He/she meets someone he/she likes better than you?
- ▶ He/she decides he/she can't commit?
- ▶ He/she receives an unexpected transfer to another part of the country or world, and he/she can't pass up the opportunity?

Strong relationships stand up to strong forces of change. Weak relationships crumble in a slight breeze. Nonetheless, people in good relationships still agonize over how future events might impact the viability of that relationship. They fret that something will cause their lover to leave them, or they agonize over what might happen if the other person changes in some unforeseen way.

As we learned in Chapter 3, all these what-ifs serve a purpose, as worry keeps us from feeling powerless. If we fret about the unthinkable, maybe we will have prevented the unthinkable from coming to pass. Of course, sometimes our worst fears are realized even when we've spent hours, days, or weeks dwelling on them. We all speculate about the future occasionally; if this is done in moderation, it can serve as the starting point to prepare and plan for future events. That's fine. But this Truth is about energy, and when we spend too much of our time and emotion creating these what-if scenarios and allowing them to consume us, then we'll have done so to no good purpose. As we Florida residents say about hurricanes, "prepare for the worst but hope for the best." We plan to manage an approaching storm, but we can neither stop the storm nor control it. Therefore, it's a waste of energy to fall apart or become overwhelmed and unable to think about or do anything else. Preparation, on the other hand, is a good use of available energy.

Worries about the future can assume all sorts of frightening forms. For instance, Dana was charged with a DUI after being pulled over with a blood alcohol level of .11 percent. The inconvenience of temporarily losing her license, the public shame and embarrassment of having her name in the newspaper for drunk driving, and the financial consequences of the arrest all proved to be quite stressful for Dana. Her attorney recommended that she seek professional counseling. Dana, an otherwise intelligent, competent, and attractive 32-year-old woman, lived in a self-created catastrophic future. She forecasted a court scene in which the judge would take away her license indefinitely. She fantasized about a work career where people would not promote her because of her DUI. She imagined that she would lose friends and forfeit potential dates because she had decided to quit drinking and would no longer be the life of the party. Dana spent the bulk of her energy every day predicting a miserable and unsuccessful future, much to the destruction of her present. Her work suffered, her social life ground to a halt, and she derived little pleasure from activities she once enjoyed.

I told Dana that even though I didn't know what the judge might decide, I could guarantee her that the judge wouldn't allow her to live the last six weeks of her life over again. She would only get one chance to live her life; it would be best not to waste it worrying about what might come to pass. Another patient, Emily, presented with severe anxiety. When she discussed her children, the anxiety was so intense it made me wonder what really frightened her. After several sessions of reassuring her that she was doing all she could do and the rest was not hers to control, Emily's real issue emerged. During her junior year in high school, a complete stranger had abducted her from a park and sexually violated her. Though she had not repressed (blocked out) the incident, she lived in a state of heightened anxiety spending her emotional energies on the fear that "something bad" would happen to her children. After all, it had happened to her. What kind of a mother would she be if she didn't worry about potential harm coming to her children?

As you'll see in Chapter 10, people like Emily can heal from their traumas so they do not invest their daily allotment of energy reliving their past by worrying about the future. In one of his clinical seminars as a Johns Hopkins University faculty member, Dr. David Edwin put it best when he said, "If I have one foot stuck in the past and one foot stuck in the future, I never have the ability to live in today" (Edwin, 1999).

Whining About the Uncontrollable Aspects of Life

A third category of nonproductive expenditure of energy is complaining about things that cannot be changed. Our practices are in southwest Florida so it is not uncommon for people to enter the office complaining about the weather or the traffic. This is understandable as people have just come from outside where they may have had to brave the elements or sit in bumper-to-bumper traffic during rush hour in the tourist season. Nonetheless, to spend a lot of time and energy on these inconveniences of life is wasteful, especially because the person sitting in the office is now in a dry, climate-controlled environment with no traffic in sight. To spend mental energy whining about the traffic or the heat isn't productive. Even worse, by focusing on or replaying the miserable ride, they continue wallowing in their negativity.

Debbie waited until she was 50 to get married. She claimed to have finally met a man that she "didn't find irritating." Unfortunately, after several blissful years of matrimony, Debbie did identify an annoying characteristic in her husband, Jesse; he didn't always put her first in communications with his family. An easy-going, peace-at-all-cost kind of guy, Jesse was inclined to allow his family a little more slack than Debbie was comfortable with. They stayed too long on visits and encroached too much on Jesse and Debbie's personal business. Debbie interpreted Jesse's inability to set appropriate boundaries with his parents as proof positive he didn't love her enough. She remained fixed on Jesse's and his family's behavior, complaining constantly to friends about the latest "outrage." She couldn't believe that his family just dropped in without calling first. She also found it hard to believe that they enjoyed watching so many sporting events on television and that Jesse joined them in this activity. She found it outrageous that they liked to eat meat for most meals despite the fact they were all somewhat overweight, and that Jesse, who normally ate healthfully, became a carnivore in their presence. She had a list of whines a mile long, and she recited them with a passion.

On the surface, Debbie's whining might have seemed harmless. In fact, it was alienating her friends who didn't want to hear about it; and it was driving a wedge between Jesse and Debbie. At first, he had understood and accepted the problems she had with his family. He had tried to change his communication style to accommodate her objections, but that didn't stop Debbie's whining about things that he told her were beyond their control. "That's just the way they are," he told her, but she acted as though complaining about his family could control them.

Eventually, Debbie came to understand this Truth. She realized that she needed to accept that she disliked this aspect of Jessie—that she thought he gave his family too much leeway—and that it was okay that she disliked how he was with his family. It didn't mean she disliked *him*. More to the point, she realized that Jesse's family was part of the package, and that if she wanted Jesse (which she did), she had to accept a small dose of his family every so often. Once she came to this acceptance, she felt much better, both emotionally and physically. Freed from thinking and talking all the time about something out of her control, she was able to concentrate on things that really mattered and which she could do something about.

Psychologists tell us that focus equals energy—where a person chooses to turn his or her thoughts, his or her energy will follow. To spend a lot of the day's energy thinking about the stubbornness of a former spouse or the selfishness of a neighbor is wasteful unless that focus solves a problem.

Vanessa is a recently divorced woman who shares custody of a 3-year-old with her ex-husband. The voice-mail messages and the exchanges, when the child is passed from one parent to the other, are often heated and ugly. The contact that Vanessa has with her ex actually totals less than an hour per week, including the time allotted for listening to his long-winded voicemails. Ironically, the amount of time she spends thinking about him, rehearsing her next conversation with him, and replaying their previous discussions is far more significant. In fact, Vanessa spends a large part of a given day's waking energy obsessing about their conflict. She continuously focuses on his negative attitude and off-putting behaviors, even though she recognizes that he's a good parent and his attitude and behaviors aren't being directed at their child. As a result of her obsessing, Vanessa, a teacher, has become much less effective in the classroom; she's more likely to have her students open a book and read than to teach them.

Patty is dating someone she refers to as "a sexist pig." Still, with her role as mother/fixer in relationships, this was a typical choice for her. As their relationship has moved forward, Patty has become increasingly frustrated that her boyfriend continues to disrespect her. She complains constantly about his behavior—both to him and to others—but nothing has changed except that Patty is becoming increasingly unhappy. It turns out that Patty has always complained about her boyfriends. She has always chosen men who have significant problems, and she has always taken on the role of trying to help change them for the better. Almost without exception, she chooses guys for their potential rather than for who they are in the present. Then she feels exhausted, not only from the futile effort of trying to change them but also from all the complaining she does about them. She can't control them, but she is compelled to talk for hours about how horrible they are, as if this whining might somehow control the uncontrollable.

Jonathan tells his therapist at every single session that he hates his boss. He hates the way his boss talks to him condescendingly; how his boss is getting rich from his hard work; how his wife loves and adores his boss. And here's the corker: Jonathan's boss is his father-in-law! It's as if his brain is a bare bulb and his boss is a moth constantly circling around it. Jonathan hasn't figured out what he wants to do about his situation at work. He doesn't know whether he wants to continue to work for his father-in-law or go into business for himself. He hasn't learned to accept his wife's closeness to her parents as he wasn't close to either of his. Jonathan fills this limbo of uncertainty with obsessive thoughts about a father-in-law boss whom he has no control over.

Jonathan is annoyed when his therapist notes the irony of spending the bulk of his daily allotment of mental energy obsessing about the person he hates the most. It's as if he's taking his paycheck and spending the bulk of it supporting the cause he hates the most. Or to state it another way, Jonathan is providing his father-in-law with free rent in his head! Jonathan needs to create a plan that will help him stop whining about his father-in-law. To that end, he should consider leaving his father-in-law's business and start his own company or find another job. Alternatively, he might also find a way to accept his father-in-law for the man he is and flourish in his current position. A third option would be for Jonathan to bargain for the changes he desires at work and reach an agreement he can live with. Jonathan needs to resolve his situation in a way that will release his energy and take back control of his head. Until he accomplishes that, he is in danger of wasting the bulk of his emotional energy fixating on the character flaws of his boss—flaws that he cannot fix. We tend to say in therapy that bitterness, resentment, and vengefulness are emotions that poison the vessel that carries them. In this case, you can hear the resentment and anger that consumes Jonathan's daily life.

Using Our Energy Rationally

This Truth guides our expenditure of mental energy as well as what we do with our time. You would think we would know better than to waste this energy on whining, worrying, and wishing, but we don't. We get caught up in the heat of the moment, the complexity and chaos of issues we're facing at any given time. As a result, we invest unwisely. Anything from a traumatic childhood experience to a head-spinning dilemma can cause us to try to fix the past, fret about the future, and agonize over the uncontrollable. On the other hand, if we follow this Truth, we can focus our energy on what matters. It suggests that we should learn to think and act rationally, to solve real problems, to focus on goals where our thoughts and actions can make a difference. Easier said than done, perhaps, but it can be done if you keep reminding yourself what your energy is and is not for. To that end, here are three energy investment corollaries of our Truth:

1. **Accept the things that you are powerless to control.** This is the mantra of Alcoholics Anonymous and other 12-step programs. In these programs, participants accept that they are "powerless over people, places, and things." The acceptance of this belief is much more conducive to peace of mind than anxiety and resentment. This doesn't mean that you should become a passive observer of your life. It simply means that it's better to recognize your lack of control over everything except your own thoughts and actions. To implement this concept, keep asking yourself if a problem or an issue you're facing is within your control. What do you need to think about in order to make a decision or take action? How can you have a positive impact on the outcome of a situation? What thought patterns and actions will have absolutely no impact on the situation?

2. **Use your energy to promote positive outcomes rather than dwell on negative mindsets.** For instance, instead of worrying

about your child's college exam to the point of nausea, consider the following options: 1) send her a positive e-mail stating how proud you are of her, 2) pray for her (research suggests that prayer actually works!), and 3) bake and mail her favorite dessert to communicate your love and admiration. The same energy required to worry yourself sick can be used to help your child. You can't do anything to ensure that she'll do well on her exam, but you can do something that makes her feel good about herself and supported no matter what her grade turns out to be.

3. **Monitor your changing energy investment.** Just as it's important to reevaluate your financial portfolio regularly, you also need to keep track of changes in how you invest your time. Create a daily energy chart that you fill out once a month. Divide this chart into the following categories: wishing the past was different; worrying about the future; and whining about the uncontrollable aspects of life; and thinking and behaving in ways that enable you to have an impact. At the end of each month, estimate how your time and energy was spent. Ideally, the wishing, worrying, and whining hours will be in the minority, and the positive thoughts and behaviors in the majority. By keeping this chart, you automatically make yourself more aware of how you are apportioning your energy. This awareness should make you much more vigilant about not wasting your energy and putting it to good use.

If you find yourself struggling to invest your energy wisely, don't worry about it. Instead, do something positive, such as any of the following exercises.

Exercises

Exercise 1—Negative to Positive

Focusing your energy on positive, attainable goals is difficult because of the "large purple elephant" reflex. This reflex comes into play when you tell yourself not to dwell on some traumatic past event, but then your mind perversely focuses on that event. Try this experiment: Close your eyes tightly and try not to think of a large, purple elephant. The odds are, that's exactly the image that came to mind. You can't tell your brain what not to focus on, but you can use this negative focus to catalyze a positive focus. This exercise demonstrates how.

List the negatives that you want to avoid, and then positively rephrase them. To help you get started, we've provided some examples of an energy-draining negative, followed by the energy-promoting positive:

Incorrect: Don't hit my golf ball into the water trap that is 75 yards in front of me.

Correct: Stay relaxed. I am confident that when using my 5-iron, the ball will travel 150 yards in flight and land in the fairway.

Incorrect: I am sick and tired of my teacher harassing me about finishing my homework, being to class on time, and other annoying stuff.

Correct: I can't control my teacher's behavior, but I can choose to do what's best for my long-term goals—apply myself, give myself enough time to do my projects, and study and prepare so that I can get to college.

Incorrect: I'm not going to show I care for my spouse as long as he/she seems to be detached.

Correct: I am going to hold myself up to the highest standards in this relationship. If my spouse seems cold, I don't have to follow suit; I can be a better person.

Incorrect:

I don't _____

I need to stop _____

I shouldn't _____

I can't _____

Correct:

My real desire is _____

I want _____

My goal is _____

I can _____

Exercise 2—The *Seinfeld* Solution

In one episode of the popular TV sitcom *Seinfeld*, Jerry tells George that if every decision he makes in life is wrong, he should do the opposite. Identify one negative thought, behavior, or pattern that has lasted a long time—one in which you dwell on the past, fret about the future, or whine about what can't be controlled. Now imagine doing the opposite, and then finish the following sentences:

Instead of expending emotional energy on _____

_____

I'm going to spend this energy on the opposite, which is _____

_____

As a result, I find that now I have more time to _____

_____

Before, I used to spend a lot of time thinking about_____

_____

Now, my thoughts often focus on _____

_____

Before, I used to spend a lot of my time doing _____

_____

Now, I spend much more time doing _____

_____

As a result of spending my energy differently, I now feel _____

_____

Exercise 3—Energy Reallocation

This activity is designed to help you recognize where your energy goes so that you can reallocate it in a more emotionally healthy way.

Past: Identify three circumstances in your life that left you feeling angry, bitter, resentful, jealous, or envious, and identify three instances when dwelling on these emotions interfered with achieving your goals.

_____

_____

_____

_____

Future: Identify three future concerns that consume you or cause you worry now. Make sure these concerns are recurring, long lasting, and distressing.

_____

_____

_____

_____

_____

Beyond your control: Identify three life or work situations that cause you great anxiety but that you cannot change.

_____

_____

_____

_____

Now use what you've learned about energy to reallocate this resource by completing the following three sentences:

Past: Instead of fixating on anger, resentment, and shame from the past, I will now focus on

_____

_____

_____

_____

_____

Future: Instead of worrying constantly about some negative event on the horizon, I will turn my attention to

_____

_____

_____

_____

_____

Beyond my control: Instead of trying to influence a person or a situation over which I have no control, I'm going to concentrate on what I can do to

_____

_____

_____

_____

_____

Chapter 7

Our Relationships Depend on Self-Empowerment and Not on Enabling Others

Question: *How many psychologists does it take to change a light bulb?*

Answer: *Only one—but the light bulb really has to want to change.*

We grasp this Truth intellectually, but our behaviors show that we don't really get it. We may acknowledge to ourselves that we can't force people to change, yet we still nag our spouse for not being sufficiently ambitious and keep reminding our kids that they better study "or else." Why do we invest so much energy in trying to alter the behavior of the people we care for? Why don't we understand that doing so not only doesn't help the other person change but may even harm the relationship? Let's take the case of the husband who hates how his wife is always late for events that he considers important. When she is tardy for his company's annual business dinner or causes them to miss the opening of a play he was looking forward to seeing, he responds by giving her the silent treatment, making sarcastic comments to her, belittling her in front of others, lecturing her about the virtues of being prompt, and/or threatening to stop attending certain functions with her.

Now think of all the things you do to manipulate others to behave differently. Do you nag, lecture, beg, plead, scold, cajole, compare, scare, insult, threaten, punish? Why would you resort to such desperate tactics?

After all, you know that you don't have the power to change people. They have to want to change. In fact, you probably have ample evidence that this is so. You may have threatened, belittled, or berated someone about being late, but it hasn't had much impact except to make this person angry at you and resentful at your attempts to control him or her. You know your tactics aren't working, but still you persist in using them. What's going on? To answer this question, we need to examine how people respond to our ineffective tactics.

Temporary Power Over Others Seems Better Than No Power at All

By chiding, cajoling, and yelling at others, you can alter behavior patterns—temporarily. A frightened child will stop teasing his little brother as long as his angry dad is around. A scolded husband may pick up his dirty dishes from the living room for a while. If she feels threatened, a tardy spouse may be ready on time for the next event. Manipulative behaviors are like alcohol and some drugs: they work in the short term to alleviate a problem, but they don't change the person or address the underlying condition. As long as they alleviate short-term suffering, they become repeated behaviors.

Let's say Joan is furious with her husband, Robert, because he spends money in excess of their budget. She has reached the point where she threatens to leave him if he continues his irresponsible spending. Even though Joan knows these threats will have no long-term efficacy, she continues to make them because they: 1) release her anger and the catharsis feels good; 2) cause Robert to apologize in response to her threats (he sometimes makes temporary changes in his spending habits); and 3) foster the illusion of power and control over his behavior. Invariably, Roberts resumes his overspending when things calm down.

The impulse to change a loved one's behavior is almost irresistible in certain circumstances, especially when doing nothing seems to invite dire consequences. This is a common response when it comes to parents and misbehaving children. For example, Tim and Betsy are involved in a power struggle with their middle school–aged son, Jason. They have graduate degrees, are successful in their chosen careers, and are very invested in their son's education. He is quite aware of their passion for education and how much power he has over them when he messes up in school. Tim and Betsy don't enjoy feeling powerless so they use the best technique they know to control him—disapproval of his study habits. This tactic is not only unproductive; it is counterproductive, and it certainly doesn't motivate Jason to try harder in school. He spites them for criticizing him by studying even less than he did before, by skipping classes, and by blowing off assignments. Tim and Betsy are smart people who recognize that Jason is rebelling against their continuing efforts to get him to take school seriously, so why do they persist? Because their efforts allow them to feel some sense of power and control over their son, even though it is illusory. They can no more browbeat Jason into being a better student than they can convince him to grow a foot taller.

Here's an extreme case that illustrates our propensity to try to convince people to change or demand that they change, why these tactics don't work, how they hurt rather than strengthen relationships. Denise is married to Charlie, a practicing alcoholic. He keeps drinking despite warnings from his physician that he won't live another six months unless he changes his behavior. Denise has experimented with various tactics to persuade him to curb his drinking. She's kicked him out of the house, only to take him back; she's negotiated to have him drink only outside of the house; she's made him promise to drink only beer; and she's demanded that he hand over his entire paycheck to her so she could control his purchases of alcohol. Not surprisingly, he's still drinking, and Denise is more frustrated than ever and frightened that she may bury her husband before he turns 40. Just as troubling, Denise's responses to Charlie's drinking have driven a wedge between them. Denise is angry and frustrated over Charlie's broken promises, and Charlie resents that Denise believes she can tell him what to do.

Denise would benefit from Al-Anon, a self-help program designed to assist people who love someone addicted to alcohol. Founded on the same principles as Alcoholics Anonymous (AA), Al-Anon emphasizes a "detach with love" model that teaches its members to take their focus off the alcoholic's drinking and on themselves instead. That is, the alcoholic's partner is taught to think about the three Cs: "I didn't **cause** the drinking problem; I can't **cure** the problem; so I must learn to **cope** effectively with the problem." Of course, this is easier said than done. The thesis of the program is that as the alcoholic is powerless over alcohol, the partner, or codependent, is powerless over the alcoholic's drinking. Powerlessness over others' behavior is tough to accept, but it's also critical in helping people address their problems and challenges. As recited in AA, we are powerless over people, places, and things.

Admitting your powerlessness doesn't mean you are powerless over yourself, your reactions to people, or what you are willing to invest in or endure in your relationships. The Truth is that self-empowerment, rather than enabling others, is the key to healthy relationships. If you focus on yourself and what you can do, you can have an indirect but significant impact on the people you care about. The reality is that you can only control yourself, and if you fail to express this fact through your behavior, you will be choosing to act in a way that is counterproductive.

Four Self-Empowerment Tactics

Again, this Truth may feel counterintuitive at first since your natural impulse is to try to save someone who is drowning, especially when you care deeply about that someone. You want to threaten, cajole, manipulate, and criticize in an attempt to get this person to change. Once you recognize that this won't work, you will need to consider effective alternatives. Fortunately, there is a four step method that focuses on self-empowerment. When you follow these steps, you'll find that the other person will be more likely to be responsive to your needs, more aware of his or her own issues, and more motivated to change in a positive way.

1. Express feelings appropriately. Take full responsibility for yourself by talking about how you feel in the first person: "I feel hurt when you call me worthless"; "I am embarrassed by arriving late at parties"; "I am frightened for your safety when you drive under the influence"; "I feel disappointed when you agree to mow the lawn after school and don't." Think in terms of "I" statements. Share with the other person the effect that his or her behavior has on you, as opposed to "you are lazy," "you are a liar," or "you are your father's son, aren't you?" These are not expressions of feelings. They are verbal putdowns/abuse. Even if you phrase your criticisms politely or qualify them—"you are trying to spare my feelings, but you're still being deceptive" or "you should know better than to challenge your teacher"—you're still making the mistake of enabling others to maintain power over you.

2. Make a specific request. Instead of issuing threats or demands and communicating how much power the other person has, try using your own power by making emotion-based requests. This isn't about constant complaining or whining, but expressing your feelings in request form. For instance: "I am so hurt by your decision to end the relationship. I wish you would reconsider marital counseling"; "I am frightened about the possibility of your failing school this year; I'd like you to make your grades more of a priority"; "I am ready to be in a committed relationship, so I'd like us to be monogamous"; or "I am hurt by the names you call me, so I'd like it if you stopped." By linking a request to an expression of feeling, you are clearly identifying that the behavior of another is adversely affecting how you feel, and by their changing that behavior, you are much more likely to feel better. You're not judging and you're not telling the other person how you think he or she should act. You're simply stating how you feel and requesting a specific action that relates to your feeling.

3. Set boundaries for yourself. In a later chapter, we'll talk in greater detail about how to set boundaries in all areas of life. Here, though, it's about marking off your turf. You're communicating your power over a well-defined and reasonable area of your life: "I don't allow smoking in my car" is a personal boundary. "We charge a 5-percent penalty for accounts not paid in full after the 15th" is a common business boundary. A speed limit is a legal boundary. You're entitled to set reasonable limits on behaviors that impact you. If you tell your spouse, "You can't invite any of your friends or family to our house," you're probably setting an unreasonable boundary.

John Wooden, the legendary basketball coach at UCLA, ran a tight ship for his Bruins. He insisted that all of his ballplayers be clean-cut for the duration of the basketball season. One year, on the first day of practice, the team's superstar and first team All American player showed up with long hair. When Wooden reminded him of the team code for players, the star announced defiantly that he liked his hair, and that Wooden didn't have the right to tell him how to wear it. "You're right," said Wooden. "I don't. I just have the right to set rules for my team. I want you to know I fully understand your feelings. And we're going to miss you." The player was back in practice the next day with a haircut.

Leo Buscaglia, a very popular author and former professor at the University of Southern California, tells this story about how he was first introduced to the concept of boundaries. As a young man, Leo was gallivanting through Europe, enjoying his newfound independence from his parents. After some time abroad, he had all but run out of money. He had to act quickly, so he decided to alert his mother about his financial woes in the most inexpensive means possible—Western Union. He sent the following telegram to his mother:

> Mama:
>
> Starving.
>
> Felice

His mother reportedly reflected on her son's telegram for a full day before deciding that this response made the most sense:

> Felice:
>
> Starve.
>
> Mama

Leo learned later that his mother's telegram was a very difficult but important way for her to help him become an independent adult. He blesses her to this day for being wise enough to set a boundary that contributed significantly to his maturation.

Other examples of boundaries include:

- ▶ "There will be no dessert served until you make a reasonable attempt at your vegetables."
- ▶ "I will not sleep with you until I have your word that this relationship is monogamous."

▶ "If you continue to arrive late for work, I will dock your pay a half hour per incident."

▶ "I choose not to be yelled at. I will leave the room if you continue to yell at me."

4. Take proper care of yourself. You gain power when you do what is necessary to enforce your boundaries. In other words, to protect yourself, you make sure you don't issue empty warnings but take actions that back up your boundaries. A speed limit is all but useless unless drivers know that troopers with radar guns are patrolling nearby. Payment deadlines are ignored without the penalty. Boundaries need teeth. So do the people who set them.

You cannot control another person, change him or her or cure his or her behavior. But you can call the police if he hits you, leave the room if she yells, or remove the computer from your teenager's room if he is found on adult sites. You can terminate relationships built on a foundation of deception. You can choose not to sleep in the same bed with your husband when he's been drinking. You can stop dating a guy until he quits lying around the house all day and shows he's serious about getting a job and pursuing a career. You can quit a job if your boss ignores your request that he stop being verbally abusive.

Although you cannot change, control, or cure another person, you can take care of yourself. This is a powerful capacity, and we would encourage you to use it, even if doing so makes you fearful or sad or costs you a relationship or a job. Taking care of yourself helps you gain self-respect. Without boundaries and the power behind them, you allow others to take advantage of you while teaching them that you accept this behavior. The Al-Anon word for this is *enabling*, the aiding of a person to do something unhealthy for him- or herself and others. Educators Jim Fay and David Funk emphasize the "love and logic" approach as an enabling preventative. This approach means making sure of the following three "ifs": if you know what is expected, if you have shared what is expected, and if you have expressed the rewards and consequences. In other words, if you are aware of these things, you don't have to overreact emotionally trying to manipulate the other person, but can enforce the consequences already established.

Enabling Makes You Weak When You Need to Be Strong

Relationships need to be egalitarian to be successful, but when you enable someone, you give that person all the power and lose your own. Enabling can be a confusing concept to people who feel they're simply helping others in need. We've had patients tell us that they knew their spouse, friend, or child was under a burden of some sort, and their behavior was designed to ease that burden. So how do you know the difference between enabling and easing a burden? Let's start out with the following song lyrics, sung to the tune of "That's Amore":

> *If you call him in sick*
> *When he's drinking with Rick*
> *That's enabling.*
> *If you're paying her bills*
> *While she's living for thrills,*
> *That's enabling.*

If your adult son is working two jobs and you know he spends money responsibly, you are merely easing his burden when you lend him money to help him afford a larger home for his family. If your spouse asks you to call her mother and make an excuse as to why she can't take her shopping that evening, and you know your spouse generally deals directly with her mom but is under a lot of pressure that day, doing what she asks is probably helping. To differentiate between helping and enabling, here is a good rule of thumb: If you are doing something for someone that he or she could or should be doing for him- or herself, you are probably enabling. When you enable another person, you prevent him or her from experiencing the consequences of his or her actions and learning from them, growing, and changing.

Here's another way to evaluate your behavior. If the other person is doing all he or she possibly can but he or she still needs assistance, then you're probably helping. True helpers generally feel good about their contributions, whereas enablers feel resentful. Helpers feel appreciated, but enablers feel used. Helpers believe they can count on the other person to reciprocate, but enablers believe that giving is a one-way street. Here is another rule of thumb to help you assess your relationship behaviors: Whenever you are working harder on someone else's life than he or she is, you are more than likely enabling. If you are working harder on funding your child's schooling than he or she is on the academics, what is he or she learning? It isn't engineering or finance, literature or philosophy—it's that the only consequences to underachieving will be absorbed by you.

To reiterate, you can't change other people; any change must take place within you. This is the key to maintaining and strengthening relationships. You evolve in a positive direction and your changes impact the other person positively. But how do you know if you are truly ready to change? If you recall our discussion of an earlier Truth, we noted that it's easier to stay stuck in resentment than it is to muster the courage to change yourself. To overcome this resistance to change and create strong relationships in your life, you need to understand the process by which human beings typically affect changes in themselves.

How to Change Yourself and Become Empowered

According to psychologists Drs. Joseph Prochaska and Richard DiClemente in their work on personal change, people move along a continuum of five stages in the change process:

Stage 1:   Pre-contemplative—the time before we are even considering change or when we are resistant to changing.

Stage 2:   Contemplative—when we become aware of the need for a modification and weigh the pros and cons of changing behaviors. There is no plan of action yet, but we understand that alteration would be beneficial.

Stage 3:   Preparation—when we decide to take positive action toward change. This is when the planning for constructive change begins.

Stage 4:   Action—when we actually change, pursuing healthier and more productive behaviors.

Stage 5:   Maintenance—when we have been in the change process for at least three months. The goal here is to continue moving forward and prevent relapse.

Think about where you are in this change process. Have you moved beyond just thinking about changing how you deal with a key person in your life? Have you decided you're definitely going to do things differently the next time you see him or her? Have you actually implemented your plan of action—talked about how you feel relative to the other person's behavior rather than criticize, for instance? Finding your place on the continuum is important, as many people become stuck in the early stages and never actually do anything different.

Prochaska and DiClemente found that of the participants who did not change, 40 percent were in the pre-contemplative stage; another 40 percent were in the contemplative stage; and the final 20 percent were in the preparation stage. Your goal should be to identify where you might be stuck and then, with the knowledge of these stages in mind, make an effort to move through each stage until you reach action and maintenance. You can conflate this change model with the four steps of self-empowerment. The first step is to express feelings appropriately, so you could start out by contemplating why you need to change the way you deal with another person and then prepare for making a change, for example. This systematic approach helps you translate self-empowerment theory into action.

Recall Charlie and Denise, and how Denise is concerned that her alcoholic husband is only months away from death if he continues to drink. All of her efforts so far have been in vain. She cannot make him stop drinking, but she can use the four steps of self-empowerment and change how she relates to him. Rather than try to control the types and amount of alcohol he drinks, lecture, plead, or threaten, Denise can express her feelings in the first person: "I love you very much. I am frightened to lose you, especially if you drink yourself to death. I am saddened by your decision to keep drinking." Second, she can make her requests known to Charlie: "I want you to go into residential rehab for alcoholism to help you get sober." Third, she can set boundaries: "I will not live with you if you continue to drink. I will leave if you do not enter rehab. I will not watch you destroy yourself with alcohol. I can't make you stop, but I will not be party to your continued drinking. Call me when you make your decision." Fourth, she must take care of herself or she'll lose credibility with Charlie.

She must follow through and enforce her boundaries by absolutely refusing to be in his presence when he's drinking and, if necessary, by leaving him if he continues to drink.

If Denise takes all four steps, Charlie is more likely to "hit bottom" and demonstrate the willingness to confront his problem and get help. By making changes in how she deals with her spouse and indirectly catalyzing Charlie's decision to stop drinking, Denise is asserting her own power. Ultimately, this is how Denise will improve her relationship with Charlie and maintain a healthy relationship.

Self-empowerment can be a bit tricky to put into practice, so let's do some exercises that will help you implement this Truth in your life.

Exercises

Exercise 1—Assess Your Enabling Tendencies

Think of the person in your life you're most often frustrated with. Consider how you interact with this person when you're frustrated and how you attempt to change or influence his behavior. We've listed various common tactics people use to leverage a response in others. Find the one or ones that best describe your approach and note specifically what you say to this person:

1. Sarcasm

   _____

   _____

   _____

2. Guilt trips

   _____

   _____

   _____

3. Threats

_____

_____

_____

4. Avoidance

_____

_____

_____

5. Comparison ("Why can't you be more like John or Joan?")

_____

_____

_____

6. Volume (shouting)

_____

_____

_____

7. Silent treatment

_____

_____

_____

Other _____

_____

_____

Exercise 2—Practice Expressing Your Feelings

This exercise is simple; try to communicate your feelings directly using "I" statements. Make the person from the previous exercise the object of these statements.

I feel _____

when you _____

I feel _____

when you _____

I feel _____

when you _____

Exercise 3—The ASSERT Formula

This is a formula you can use to express your feelings and make requests without criticism, rancor, and other negative behaviors. Self-empowerment can take place without disempowering others if you follow the ASSERT formula:

A: Gain the **Attention** of the other person.

S: Do this **Soon** after the problem occurs.

S: Be **Specific** about the behavior. Don't attack the other person.

E: Use "I statements" to discuss the **Effect** of this problem from your point of view.

R: Offer a new **Response** or alternative way of dealing with this problem.

T: Define the new **Terms** of the relationship. Share with this person how using the new response/alternative behavior will have a positive effect on your relationship.

Now, apply the ASSERT formula to a relationship in your life. Write what you would do and say at each step:

A: How will you gain the attention of this person?

_____

_____

_____

S: How soon after the incident that you need to address will you have a discussion?

_____

_____

_____

S: What specific behavior will you talk about?

_____

_____

_____

_____

E: What are the effects of this behavior on you?

_____

_____

_____

_____

R: What is the response you want from this person?

_____

_____

_____

_____

T: What are the new terms of the relationship once the new response is
   in effect?

_____

_____

_____

_____

Exercise 4—Boundary Enforcement Options

If your spouse, child, significant other, parent, or friend chooses to continue unhealthy, unacceptable behavior and defies the boundaries you've set, have options ready to enforce your boundaries. In this exercise, describe the boundary-crossing behavior, and then list three enforcement options:

If my spouse/significant other continues to _____

_____

I will _____

I can _____

I am ready to _____

If my acquaintance/friend continues to _____

_____

I will _____

I can _____

I am ready to _____

If my family member continues to _____

_____

I will _____

I can _____

I am ready to _____

Chapter 8

Ego Boundaries Protect
Us From Rejection,
Insult, and Intimidation

Not one drop of my self-esteem depends on your approval.

—Ray Charles

Everyone is kneaded out of the same dough but not baked in the same oven.

—Yiddish Proverb

Parade magazine's June 10, 2007 issue asked this question: "Why are beauties like Halle Berry, Christie Brinkley, and Sienna Miller cheated on by their partners?" And more to the point, if these ladies aren't able to keep their lovers happy and satisfied, what chance do the rest of us have? Just how beautiful does a woman have to be to ensure fidelity in her partner? *Parade*'s "Hollywood Relationship Guru," Kathryn Alice, addresses this question by writing that "partners cheat due to their own problems—anger, boredom, jealousy, sexual addiction—not due to something lacking in their women." Ms. Alice suggests that the behavior of the cheater reflects only on the cheater, and not on the value or desirability of the person cheated on. So how do these women protect themselves from the problems of the people to whom they're married? More to the point, how do we protect ourselves from the mean words and hurtful actions of those we care about or work with? The answer is ego boundaries.

Knowing Where You Stop and the Other Person Begins

A boundary is a line that separates something from something else. The word *ego* means "self," so an *ego boundary* is an awareness of where we end and another person begins. Psychologists also call this *ego differentiation*. Everything that you think, feel, say, or do is a statement about you. Everything that I think, feel, say, or do is a statement about me. Therefore, how I treat you is much more a statement about me than it is about you. If I'm kind to you, that only testifies to my capacity and willingness to be kind. If I'm condescending to you, again, that testifies to my capacity and willingness to condescend.

The Rorschach test is a psychological instrument that affords the test-taker the opportunity to project his or her thoughts, feelings, and unique way of conceptualizing the world onto a piece of paper spattered with ink. Not coincidentally, this type of test is called a *projective test* and is designed to gain information about a person's way of processing reality from a non-specific stimulus such as a blob of ink.

Other people see each of us as those blobs of ink in that they project their perceptions upon us. This is why some people ignore us while others worship us, and why some resent us while others obsess about us. Think about the people you know best. Do any of them understand the real you? Do they have different perceptions of who you are? There is a saying that if a thousand people know you, you are a thousand different people. Everyone who knows you will think of you in their own unique way and treat you accordingly. Again, how each one treats you is a statement about who they are, not who you are! The point is that you must set up clear ego boundaries or you're going to be vulnerable to any negative (or overly positive) comment or action. It's not your problem if you have a friend who is in a bad mood and responds to your innocuous comment with a critical assault on your decency and compassion, but you make it your problem when you have not established healthy ego boundaries. The story of the five blind men makes this point clear:

Five blind men set out on separate journeys to discover for
themselves true knowledge. A wise teacher told them all
to search for a strange animal that is the source of wisdom.
They know only that this animal is called an elephant. On
their journeys, each man comes across the elephant and
begins to touch it in order to discover what the animal is
like. The first man grabs hold of the elephant's leg and
thinks that what he holds is like a tree trunk, firm and solid.
He exclaims that the elephant is like a pillar. The second
man takes hold of the elephant's ear and decides that the
elephant is like a ship's sail. The third man holds on to the
elephant's tail and says that the elephant is like a rope. The
fourth man strokes the elephant's tusk and concludes that
the elephant is smooth and sharp. And the fifth man holds
the tongue and thinks that the elephant is wet and warm.
When the five men consult each other, each has a different
version of what the elephant is like. Each has discovered
truth, but none has gathered the whole truth about the
animal, nor has any one of them discovered what gave life
to the elephant. Each one has developed a partial view of
the stimulus known as an elephant, according to his own
perceptions.

Psychologists have discovered that most external stimuli do not evoke
specific feelings in people unless there has been prior exposure and
learning. (The exception to this would be a noxious or painful stimulus—
for example, a loud noise or an electric shock.) A person without prior
knowledge of weapons encountering someone holding a gun would likely
react neutrally, whereas someone with prior exposure would react quite
differently. This also holds true in our interpersonal relations. Think
about it: You project your perceptions (based upon prior history) upon
me (a neutral stimulus) and treat me accordingly. You may think of me
as a savior, an idiot, a lust object, or an obstacle in your life. Am I any,

some, or all of these things? It doesn't matter—at least not in terms of how you relate to me—because you'll treat me according to how you perceive me.

Katie had gastric bypass surgery, a last-ditch attempt to cure her morbid obesity in the hope of transforming and lengthening her life. The bypass required a drastic change in her eating habits; virtually anything that she might have once considered a meal was now prohibited. On Thanksgiving, Katie was invited to have dinner at Joan's house, who is a friend of Katie's friend. Katie was barely able to eat more than a few bites of turkey. Joan, who didn't know Katie well, was insulted when Katie declined to try her stuffing. Joan takes great pride in her stuffing, and each year everyone raves about it. Katie tried to explain about her surgery and that she would become ill if she ate too much, but Joan chose to believe she had been insulted and refused to accept the possibility that anyone could turn down her stuffing.

Why would Joan feel insulted? For one thing, her self-esteem seems at least partially tied up in others' opinions of her and her cooking. She also lacks the ability to differentiate Katie's seeming unwillingness to eat from the quality and appeal of her stuffing. At first glance, it may sound as though Joan is unreasonable at best and unhinged at worst, but Joan's response is not dissimilar from how many of us respond to what we perceive to be rejection from others. If we don't create firm ego boundaries, we can globalize a single response, making it more meaningful than it really is. It's one thing to feel angry and resentful because someone doesn't eat your stuffing; it's something else entirely when your ego boundaries are so weak that it impacts the most important relationship in your life.

Sheila was married for 30-plus years to Bill, who was not particularly demonstrative of his love for Sheila. Still, they had a good relationship and Sheila was reasonably happy. Then Sheila met Carl. He was everything her husband wasn't—charming, flattering, and infatuated with Sheila. He thought she was beautiful and told her so. Carl visited her often at the place where she worked, sent her poetry, and spoke of nights when he would lie awake just thinking about her. Sheila left her husband for Carl and reported feeling happier than at any time in her life because she felt truly loved and adored. Carl was captivated by her and expressed it eloquently and frequently. When Sheila moved in with Carl, though, everything changed. She began to see a coldness in him that had previously gone undetected. The flowers and poetry ceased. The reservoir of compliments dried up. The affection disappeared completely. As soon as Carl had completed his conquest, Sheila was no longer a worthy prize. Sheila told him how hurt she was by his coldness, and this made him even more indifferent to her. He told her to leave, and Sheila felt ashamed, defeated, and worthless. Even worse, she couldn't move on with her life. She kept asking herself, "What is so wrong with me that Carl stopped loving me?" She lost her husband. She lost Carl. Worst of all, Sheila lost herself. She needed to start her life over as a divorced woman. However, the nagging, obsessive pain she experienced was not about loss. It was about her perception of her worthlessness and unlovable nature. "What is wrong with me?" was her refrain.

Carl's infatuation with Sheila had little to do with love. In fact, he had used the same romantic approach with other women in the past, only to dump them when they fell for him. It was all about Carl, not Sheila. It wasn't about her "worthlessness" or her "unlovable nature." However, she internalized Carl's treatment of her and it wounded her deeply. For the rest of her life she never had another romantic relationship.

Now consider Monique, who entered therapy because of problems with her boyfriend, Luke. In the initial stages of the relationship, Monique believed she had found someone she would spend her life with but things had deteriorated fast as Luke constantly disrespected her. At first, when Luke would belittle her in public, she would laugh it off or try to ignore it. His attitude also prevented Monique from engaging him in important or deep conversations. As Luke continued his rude behavior, she began to question her dreams and expectations. She accepted his negativity and convinced herself that she was somehow expecting too much.

In therapy, Monique began to realize that she had failed to create the boundaries that would protect her from *his* issues. Monique grasped that what she wanted (open communication, commitment, and respect) were not excessive demands. Luke's belittling responses to these reasonable desires was a reflection on him and his lifelong difficulties with women who weren't completely acquiescent. Monique eventually grasped that she had allowed him to bully her to a point at which she no longer was behaving according to the healthy standards of a loving relationship. As a result, she drew a figurative line around herself, one that clearly separated herself from his desire to control her, his issues with women, and his bullying behaviors. In this way, she was able to tell Luke what she considered unacceptable behavior. When he ignored her clearly communicated expectations, she ended the relationship. She didn't take his refusal to abide by her desires as a reflection on her; she had protected herself and so was able to end the relationship without remorse or self-loathing.

You Are Not Responsible for What Others Say and Do

Forgive us for belaboring this point, but people are not very adept at constructing and maintaining ego boundaries. As a result, they succumb to this "what is wrong with me" thinking based on a single incident. As therapists, we often see people who believe something is terribly wrong with them. John believes he must be inherently unlovable because his mother walked out on him and the rest of the family when he was two. Ginny feels especially ashamed and responsible because her father sexually abused her as a girl, but not (to her knowledge) her two sisters; she must have done something to be the target of his perverse desires. Larry questions his worth because his stepfather beat him daily and regularly locked him in a closet as a form of discipline.

What if you were mugged? Raped? Swindled by a phone scam artist? Betrayed by a lover or a best friend? Molested by a neighbor? Ignored by a parent? Seduced by your therapist? Insulted by your boss? Defied by your child? What do these things say about you and your worth as a person? Absolutely nothing! Someone else's behavior is not about you. You were a child, for example, who deserved to be loved—not abused or abandoned. As a lover or a friend, you did not cause your loved ones to deceive or betray you. As unfortunate and painful as they might be, these behaviors do not belong to you. They are no more yours than your neighbor's pine tree, although the needles do fall all over your yard.

If your ego boundaries are in place, however, these events won't cause you to be ashamed, sad, or fearful. Obviously, if your friend tells you he thinks you're a coward because you won't level with him, you won't feel good about it. But his harsh words don't cause you to define yourself by his accusation. You protect yourself by recognizing that what he's saying is much more about him—about his insecurities and fears—than about you. Please understand that this doesn't mean you should blame all your problems on somebody else and take on the role of innocent victim. We couldn't help our patients if we didn't assign them responsibility for their own issues in life. So what belongs to you? What is yours is what you bring to the table—your thoughts, your attitudes, your feelings, your behavior. This includes your reactions to the behavior of others. That's what belongs to you. Their behavior is about them; your reactions are about you. As we say to couples in marriage counseling, you are each 100-percent responsible for your 50 percent of the relationship.

In the previous example, Sheila's low self-esteem may have led her to display flirtatious, provocative behaviors that encouraged Carl to seduce her. Sheila is responsible for those behaviors as well as her poor self-image, but she is never responsible for Carl's mindset or his poor treatment of her once he achieved his conquest. Drawing boundaries to protect yourself from what doesn't belong to you is crucial for your mental well-being. Without these boundaries, you're vulnerable to every Carl who crosses your path. Remind yourself that you are only responsible for understanding why you do what you do and for your behavior.

Ego boundaries aren't just useful in dealing with spouses or significant others. They are also useful in parenting. Pat was not prepared for her 21-year-old daughter, Amy, to drop out of college and elope with her boyfriend—a guy that no one in the family liked. Pat was surprised by Amy's behavior. When she was growing up, Amy was the most considerate of the five children, the most respectful of her parents' rules. Where had this new behavior come from? "I must have failed her in some way," Pat moaned to her therapist. "What did I do to make her exclude us from her wedding? Didn't she realize we'd be devastated?"

Pat's situation would be difficult for most parents, but her "devastation" was more the product of her self-blame than her daughter's actions. Although Amy hadn't included any of her family in her sudden decision to drop out of school, marry, and relocate, somehow it had become Pat's fault. She had failed as a mother, not her husband as a father. In Pat's mind, she must have done something wrong to cause Amy to exclude the family from the wedding. Pat could not separate Amy's decisions from her parenting. If she had ego boundaries—if she had clearly differentiated who she was and where her responsibilities ended—she would not have been so torn up by her daughter's elopement. She would have been able to handle it maturely and sensitively, thus ensuring a continuing strong relationship with Amy.

What Part Is Yours?

Although boundaries are critical, they shouldn't serve as barriers against consensus opinions. By that we mean that if you receive the same feedback or behavioral responses from a number of people, pay attention—they might be telling you something that you should heed. We recommend that you "try on" all the feedback you receive about yourself. At the very least, evaluate the feedback, reflect on it, and determine if it's valid. Whatever seems to fit, be brave enough to own it and change when necessary. Whatever doesn't fit, put back on the rack. It's not yours. If numerous people find you annoying, for instance, you probably are. That's yours to own and change; but even if you are annoying, how others respond to you is up to them. They may like you despite being annoyed by you. They may grimace at some of the annoying things you say but show no other reaction. They may tell you that you annoy them but that they love you anyway. They may cut you off completely and send you a note that you're too annoying to be their friend. All of these reactions belong to them. It is up to you to evaluate this consensus response and determine what it means and how you want to respond to it.

To say it another way, if someone tells you that you look like a horse, you can laugh at the statement. If a second person says you look like a horse, you may decide that this is only a coincidence. If a third person says you look like a horse, it may be time to buy a saddle. Consistent feedback from others can be painful to hear, but it may be information that we need to hear. If all your friends tell you you're cheap, be brave enough to own it (and pick up the next lunch tab). If you continually hear that you have amazing hair, believe it, smile, and say thank you. If you are told that you are tone deaf by all four judges on American Idol, don't call your lawyer— call your voice teacher!

Ego boundaries allow you to put another person's irksome behavior in perspective. Think about someone in your life who does or says things that bother you. It may be your child's shyness, your husband's selfishness, your girlfriend's nagging or your boss' criticism. Whatever it is, recognizing it as originating with them, and not you, can diminish the behavior's impact on you. It doesn't make it go away, and it still may hurt, but the only things that can devastate you are the ones that you take personally. Use the Truth from the previous chapter to remind yourself that you didn't cause the behavior and can't control or cure it, so you must cope with it. Empower yourself rather than giving someone else the power to determine how you feel. Similarly, make an effort to understand where this other person is coming from. The more you understand another person, the less apt you will be to take his or her behavior personally.

You learn that when your mother is under a lot of stress at work, she tends to be short-tempered and says things she doesn't really mean. When your sister experiences stress in her marriage, she tends to withdraw from you and make you feel as if you've done something wrong. When your boyfriend feels insecure, he accuses you of being unfaithful. Your boss tends to micromanage your work when your group's results fall below the monthly target. People will do what makes sense to them, not what you prefer that they do. If you know their patterns of behavior, why not expect them to do what they tend to do instead of expecting them to do otherwise? More to the point, why not set your ego boundary so you don't let their way of acting impact you in a negative way?

Few things are more irritating to therapists than patients who miss appointments but don't call in advance to cancel. We worry that something may have happened to them. We are concerned that we may have said or done something at the last session that has caused them to stay away. Yet if we know that a patient has displayed this same behavior in the past and that this is how he or she is now, we don't need to take it personally. This understanding reduces our pain and frustration because we're not personalizing it. We don't feel that we are lousy psychologists because the patient fails to call, or conclude that his or her tardiness means that we are not worthy of respect.

To keep your boundaries clearly in place, it may help to think of your life as a movie and the people you know as characters in the movie. In a film, characters stay in character. In your own mind, you label each person: the psychopath, the good girl, the best friend, the nerd, the romantic lead, and so on. Based on these labels, you know what to expect of each person. The bully in a movie doesn't suddenly turn into the hero, and the flirtatious coworker remains flirtatious. If they do change their behaviors—which is unusual—it's usually due to a life-changing event, such as the death of a loved one or something of similar magnitude. Even in the movies, however, this 180-degree turnaround doesn't ring true. You can think of your family, friends, and work colleagues as stock characters in a movie. You can create a mental list of dominant traits, quirks, problems, and strengths that define each person, and based on this list, you can set reasonable expectations for how each person is going to act. When someone does something that offends or hurts you in some way, you can say to yourself, "That's just Chuck being Chuck." You're reminding yourself that he's staying true to his character and that his behavior has nothing to do with you.

Erin calls her mother long distance once a week and endures conversations in which her mother is hypercritical of her and her lifestyle. Erin's mom couches her disapproval in "helpful" tidbits of advice, which are neither asked for nor well-received by Erin. Erin has internalized her mother's critical observations and is caught in her mother's web of negativity. Instead of defending, negating, arguing, or hanging up crying, Erin needs to understand her mother better in order to set and enforce her boundaries. To achieve this goal, Erin was asked to make a list of the suggestions and criticisms her mother is likely to make during a conversation. During their call, Erin can then check off each forecasted item that her mother brings up. In this way, she is able to detach herself from the criticisms. By anticipating the issues her mother will raise, she gains some insight into her mother's own issues. This takes some of the sting out of her comments and helps Erin keep in mind that this is about her mom. As Erin said, "If I know mom better, I'll personalize her issues less." Erin's observation is worth repeating once again. The better you understand another person, the less you take his or her behavior personally.

The Social Black Belt

Mastering ego boundaries—understanding where you end and others begin—can help you attain a social black belt. A black belt in martial arts prepares people to protect themselves from various physical threats. Similarly, a social black belt affords protection in personal interactions. If you have such a belt, you will be able to withstand the insulter's need to insult, parrying demeaning comments with your awareness that these comments say more about the insulter than about you. Such a belt will also help you rebound from a philanderer's propensity to be unfaithful; rather than make you feel unworthy of a relationship, it will give you the courage to enter into a new and potentially better relationship. You can also depend on this belt to help you deal effectively with rejection, whether from a boss, a lover, or a friend. You recognize that this rejection is about what this person feels he or she needs to do now, and it doesn't mean that others will reject you for the same reasons.

You can expect to be rejected, insulted, mocked, and embarrassed. No matter how smart, successful, or empathetic you happen to be, others are going to hit you where it hurts. They may not even know where you're vulnerable, but somehow, they say or do something that strikes at a tender spot. You can block or at least absorb these blows if you possess a social black belt. When you recognize that this is all about the other person, you aren't hurt as much (or at all) by what this person says or does. Just as important, you gain courage and confidence when you realize you can take it. When you understand that who you are has nothing to do with what a mean-spirited boss or lover has to say about you, you lose a lot of your relationship fear. In other words, when you know that other people can't devastate you as they may have done in the past, you can release your fear and move forward with forming positive relationships.

A social black belt also equips you to do things that the socially self-conscious tend to avoid like the plague: entering a party, restaurant, or bar alone; leading a group; initiating a conversation with a complete stranger; and, yes, even mastering public speaking. In short, having a social black belt equips you to be comfortable in your own skin, wherever you are and whomever you're with.

How do you obtain such a belt? Like the martial arts belt, it requires practice—practice defining and establishing your ego boundaries. You need to work at relinquishing responsibility for the thoughts, feelings, and actions of others, always keeping in mind that people will continue to do what makes sense to them—not what is most pleasing to you. Because the social black belt is really a mindset, it may help to adopt this attitude: "I am worthwhile; I belong here and so does everyone else [in this group, family, team, and so on]; I will treat them the way I want to be treated, but I cannot control their responses to me. I am open to learning more about myself and others, and I will bravely attempt to make positive changes when necessary. Others cannot hurt me by what they say unless I endorse it. I will not live in fear of the words of others but will evaluate their responses carefully and appropriately, remembering that I am only a stimulus upon which they project themselves."

The following exercises will help you meet this goal.

Exercises

Exercise 1—Practice Differentiating

The goal of this exercise is to help you become adept at differentiating your values and beliefs from others and drawing your ego boundaries. Start out by thinking about a key person in your life and a topic that creates tension or other problems in this relationship. For instance, you and your sister may frequently argue about your choice of boyfriends. Whatever topic and person you choose, the next step is to differentiate your thoughts and feelings regarding this topic versus those of the other person. Try this exercise with one person, then do it again with another friend, work colleague, or family member.

Topic _____	You	Other (Spouse, Boss, Parent)
Value		
Belief		
History		
Expectation		
Reaction		

Topic _____	You	Other (Spouse, Boss, Parent)
Value		
Belief		
History		
Expectation		
Reaction		

Exercise 2—Cast Your Movie

This activity will help you set expectations for key people in your life, enabling you to anticipate their modus operandi and prevent their negative behaviors from crossing the boundaries you've set. Think of your life as a movie and the key people you know as the main characters. Create a cast list in which you do the following:

1. Name at least five key people in your life who will be featured in this movie.

2. Create a brief description of each of these people that defines how you expect him or her to behave (for example: brother-in-law—sarcastic, insecure, quick-witted).

3. Using the description, find the perfect word to describe the role of each person (brother-in-law: the Joker).

4. Using each person's name, label, and description, write a brief plan of how you will handle them the next time they behave in character (this can include your thoughts and behaviors).

Exercise 3—Draw the Line

To set your ego boundaries, start out by thinking about incidents in the recent past when another person's words or deeds caused you to feel ashamed, embarrassed, worthless, stupid, or hopeless. Complete any of the relevant following sentences by filling in the blanks:

When _____

    told me I was _____

    I felt ashamed because _____

    _____

When _____

    acted meanly toward me by _____

    I felt devalued because _____

    _____

When _____

    lectured me about _____

    I felt like an idiot because _____

    _____

When _____

    yelled at me at work, I felt like I was a failure because

    _____

When _____

    rejected me, I felt as if I would never have another meaningful

    relationship because _____

    _____

Now, rewrite each sentence two ways. Rewrite the second part of the sentence by describing why you won't allow the other person to dictate your feelings. For example, "When Judy told me that I embarrassed her when we went out on a date, I felt ashamed because I must be a stupid person" would be rewritten as "When Judy told me that I embarrassed her when we went out on a date, I realized that she was being hypersensitive to any critical remark I made, so I had no reason to feel ashamed." Then, rewrite the second part again by reminding yourself of how you can protect yourself against the negative feeling. For example, this same sentence could be rewritten as "When Judy told me that I embarrassed her when we went out on a date, I reminded myself that I am a compassionate, empathic person who tries hard to think of the feelings of others."

Chapter 9

You Can Trust People to Be Who They Are, Not Who You Want Them to Be

Because a man is unfaithful is no reason to leave him. You should stay with him and make sure the rest of his life is a living hell.

—Roseanne Barr

Dennis never expected his wife, Cynthia, to leave, let alone run off with his close friend. He felt crushed and humiliated by his wife's decision to move in with another man. Nevertheless, before the reality of her decision had had a chance to completely register with him, Dennis met Tiffany at a local singles bar. Before you could say Jerry Springer, Dennis was living with a virtual stranger. Okay, no big deal—yet. Not until Cynthia learned about Tiffany did she become enraged. She didn't want her husband living with some "bimbo," so she made a play to get Dennis back and kicked out Dennis's friend. Dennis went for the bait and returned to his wife for a weekend before deciding that he missed Tiffany and went back to her. Cynthia wasn't giving up easily, however; she continued to find reasons to have Dennis drop by so she could try to seduce him to stay. He visited occasionally, re-consummated his marriage, and then went back to Tiffany. These conjugal visits with his wife continued during the next few weeks.

When Tiffany caught on to what Dennis was doing, she experienced her own meltdown. She shared her story with friends and relatives, who, not surprisingly, attempted to steer her away from Dennis. Nonetheless,

Tiffany felt like she was in a competition with Cynthia—a competition she desperately wanted to win. Her strategy: to hook up with the guy with whom Cynthia originally had the affair. Her strategy didn't work, and Dennis and Cynthia decided to give it another shot. Seeking a therapist in an attempt to increase the odds of marital success, they told me that they wanted to "learn to trust one another."

Although most people do not have the baggage that this couple dragged in, establishing and building trust is a major focus of therapy. Typically, people ask, "What can you do so that he can finally be trusted?" or "Please fix her so that she becomes trustworthy." However, changing people is not within a therapist's or anyone else's power. So what do we do with people whom we can't trust? We trust them to be themselves. At the same time, we cannot trust them to be who we want them to be or who we need them to be. People do what makes sense to them, not necessarily what makes sense to us, not necessarily what makes us happy, and not necessarily what they promised they would do. If all things were equal, we would be able to trust everyone without fear of exploitation or disappointment. Unfortunately, not everyone shares our value system, beliefs, or expectations.

Types of Trust

When we think about it, we realize that we don't trust blindly or equally. We may have a great relationship with our spouse and trust him implicitly when it comes to the big things, but we may not trust him as far as we can throw him when it comes to taking out the trash. In other instances, we may trust our spouse to provide us with financial support, but we may not trust her to stop drinking to excess. In short, how we trust someone varies considerably. Here are some specific variations on trust:

- ▶ A man may trust his wife to be faithful in most circumstances, but he knows she likes tall, swarthy men similar to the first baseman on her coed softball team, so he attends every one of her games.

- ▶ A woman trusts her teenage son to refrain from using drugs, but never to baby-sit his 5-year-old sister.

▶ A man trusts his wife with all of his personal secrets, but not to drive his new Corvette.

▶ A woman trusts her husband to manage all of their financial affairs, but knows not to let him come within a mile of a casino because of his gambling problem.

The assumption in all of these examples is this: We can trust people to be who they are and do what they do. This includes continuing to do whatever they do well or not so well. We know that a guy who has cheated on his last three girlfriends is likely to cheat on his fourth. We may *want* to trust him. We may believe him when he says he's changed and will be faithful forevermore. It's possible that he means what he says, and it's possible that he will work hard to keep his promise. Yet it is difficult to trust someone to act in a way that runs counter to a long-term behavioral pattern. If we're honest with ourselves, we know what we can trust people to do—and not do.

We can't change others. If they want to change themselves, come to a new level of insight, realize their patterns and underlying needs, sustain motivation, and develop healthier patterns of behavior, they can change. But we can't make change happen, no matter how much we want to turn someone into the person we think he or she could and/or should be. The problem with implementing this Truth, however, is that our hopes and needs play havoc with our ability to trust people to be who they are. When we're so focused on another person living up to our standards or expectations, we trust them to be how we want them to be—often a big mistake.

The parent-child relationship provides ample evidence of how we fail to observe this Truth. Consider homework. Parents repeatedly ask their children, "Do you have homework tonight?" and "Is your homework done?" The answers to these questions are typically no and yes, respectively. When parents become aware that their child has not been doing his or her homework and is receiving poor grades, they are upset. Much of this upset stems from the perception of betrayal of trust: "You told us that your homework was done. You lied to us!" Parents then decide to punish the child, often by grounding him or her. They may also assume a stronger position of control over the child, perhaps by having weekly progress reports signed by the teacher and by going over homework with the child on a nightly basis.

Although there's nothing wrong with this approach in one sense, it illustrates how our expectations often supersede reality. We trust that our children will conform to what we expect of them rather than what's in their nature to do. When they act naturally and avoid taking responsibility, don't follow through, or are not accountable for their actions, we feel hurt and betrayed. We thought they were responsible (or hoped that they would magically become responsible overnight) and they proved us wrong. Although we feel betrayed, they may in fact be communicating why they act the way they do. Perhaps they just aren't interested in math and they need/want you to push them to study harder. Or perhaps they prefer practicing their guitar or playing video games. Rather than feel hurt and disrespected, we should listen to what their behavior is saying. We should recognize that no matter how much we lecture or punish them in response to their behavior, their own nature is more powerful than our harsh words and stern sanctions. We need to trust in who they are rather than in our own hopes and expectations, which may be completely out of touch with reality.

Ignoring this Truth—pretending that someone with a history of irresponsibility will suddenly become responsible—means going through life being constantly disappointed by other people. If we trust others to be who we want them to be, it is like walking outside on summer mornings in southwest Florida expecting snow. We are not wrong to want it; we're just not likely to get what we want. If we stand outside in the Florida summer, it makes sense to trust that heat and humidity will envelop us. Counting on an unlikely outcome is a set-up for failure.

When parents bring an underachieving child to see a mental health professional, the child, at first, may alter his or her behavior in some manner, presumably because of the focus on him or her and the presenting issue. After some of the initial focus is removed, however, parents are greatly disappointed when the child reverts to old, more comfortable behaviors. This doesn't mean that we should give up on children who don't do their homework. It's possible for them to change and be more diligent, but first they must internalize the importance of being a good student.

People can only be trusted to do what makes sense to them. Studying may not make sense to a homework-averse student. If a behavior surprises us, that's because we don't know our loved one as well as we thought we did. This is part of what hurts so much. Not only did this person do something we were certain he or she would never do, but now we are face-to-face with our lack of insight and knowledge about this person. Our tendency is to attribute untrustworthiness, if not maliciousness, to the loved one, rather than to recognize that the deficit lies in our own misunderstanding of the other person's motivations and behavior.

Ironically, choosing to trust someone is really about trusting ourselves. The lover may cheat again, the child may underreport the homework assignment, and the salesperson may lie, but we can trust ourselves to deal appropriately with the outcome. For example, Karen began dating Tim, a guy her friend Jill used to go out with. She had heard from Jill that Tim was a great guy—smart, successful, charming—but that he had a tendency to stray. Jill said she broke up with him because he had been seeing another woman when they were going out, and she had heard he had done the same thing to a former girlfriend. Still, Karen believed that she and Tim had something special as soon as they met. They both had a great time on their first date, and after a month, Karen began thinking about a long-term relationship. Then Tim didn't call for a week. He eventually admitted that he had been out of town seeing his ex-wife and that although they had had sex, it was more out of a sense of "nostalgia." Jill was disappointed in Tim's behavior, yet she knew exactly what she had to do. She told Tim it was over between them, and after a brief period of feeling badly about what might have been, she moved forward with her life. For the most part, she didn't mope or mourn the loss of Tim. She absolutely believed in herself and her ability to find a guy who valued her as much as she valued him. In fact, a week after their relationship ended, Jill said she rarely thought about him, and certainly didn't feel devastated by the loss. In short, Jill trusted herself. Initially, she may have hoped that Tim would become someone he was not, but this false trust in who he was ended shortly after he cheated on her.

Unfortunately, many people aren't like Jill; they trust that people will somehow magically deviate from their normal behavioral patterns. Therapists often see patients who clearly are entering into relationships in which they "know" that the other person is not to be trusted. Nonetheless, their hope for the relationship is so strong that it overwhelms their common sense. One therapist had a patient who dated a guy who lost his temper and yelled at her on their very first date. "Perfect!" the therapist exclaimed, much to her surprise. "You know everything you need to know about him on the first date. You can trust him to anger quickly and yell at you all throughout the relationship. If that's a big turn-on for you, then keep dating him because that's what's in store for the future." If this woman had been thinking clearly, she would have read the situation correctly without having to have the therapist spell it out for her. If he yelled at her on a first date when most people are on their best behavior, he probably would continue and even escalate this behavior on future dates. It doesn't take a psychologist to know that this guy has anger management problems, control issues, and possibly (woman-hating) misogynistic tendencies.

It often does take a therapist to alert people that others can be trusted to be themselves, but even therapists can't prevent people from trusting that others will become who they want them to be. In this particular situation, the woman ignored the advice of her therapist and wound up in a relationship that segued from verbally to physically abusive. As psychologists, we sometimes see patients who spend much of their adult lives trying to gain a parent's approval even though this parent never gave it to them when they were children. One patient, Jillian, talked about how she wished for approval and loving affirmation from her father but never received it. Her father traveled a lot during her childhood and her mother provided the love and attention. In school and as an adult, Jillian has enjoyed tremendous success—valedictorian of her high school class and CEO of a major organization—but her father has never acknowledged this success with so much as a "good job." Yet Jillian is desperate for it and cannot be truly happy without it—or at least that's how she has felt for years. She needs to recognize that her happiness should not be dependent on someone else's behavior. Additionally, Jillian needs to face reality rather than continue to set herself up for disappointment.

Can We Ever Trust Again?

So far it may sound as though we're advising you to be constantly on your guard for bad behavior on the part of people you care about. It may appear that we're cynical about human nature. In fact, we're neither cynical nor pessimistic about relationships; what we are is realistic. We know that if people exhibit a behavioral pattern through time they will likely continue it, no matter how fervent our trust that they'll behave in a different manner. Perhaps it would help if you considered trust from a slightly different perspective. Whether to trust someone is your choice and your issue; whether that someone *is* trustworthy is his/her responsibility and his/her issue. If your child says his homework is done, if your tenant says the check is in the mail, if your lunch date promises to make it on time the next time, it's your choice to believe it or not (with apologies to Ripley). If you recall the Truth from Chapter 5, people can choose to retract permission for doing certain things. You may have fresh evidence that this person has broken or is trying to break from his/her pattern. Although your spouse has cheated on you in the past, perhaps, through counseling and reflection, he has made a commitment not to cheat on you again.

Some people stop cheating. Some stop drinking or lying or procrastinating or hitting or yelling or shoplifting or whatever. Why? Fear of consequences, spiritual conviction, emotional maturity, therapeutic intervention, and so on. The capacity for exhibiting old behaviors is still there, but the permission is gone. How do we know if this time is the real deal, when she has told us twice before that she has quit smoking pot? And how do we know that he doesn't have a secret e-mail address, cell phone, or mailbox? What about the teenager who may only be showing us the grades and reports that will pass our inspection? How do we ever know? We don't, not for certain. But we do have a way to deal with our uncertainty and increase the odds of making a good decision about trusting other people. Let us change our pronouns to first person singular to describe the thought process that you can adapt to your own circumstances:

> Now that I know I can trust you only to be yourself, whoever that may be, I must trust myself to deal with the potential consequences of your behavior. I don't know if my tenants will damage my house—I may trust that they will not, and penalize them if they do—but I trust myself to deal with whatever happens. I don't know if my child will really do his homework if left alone, but I trust myself to respond appropriately if he does not. I don't know if my spouse will finally end her relationship with the other man, but I must trust myself to deal with the possibility that she will not. I can choose to terminate the relationship based on that fact; or, if I choose to continue to invest in this person, I ultimately trust myself to cope with the real possibility that history will repeat itself. If I can't handle finding out one more time that she has been unfaithful, I may consider getting out of the marriage. Because I don't know that she can be trusted and I have decided that I cannot trust myself to withstand the infidelity, I may need to remove myself from this toxic situation.

In line with the Truth about self-empowerment in Chapter 7, this kind of self-talk shifts the power from the other person to you. It raises your consciousness that people can disappoint you and won't fulfill your expectations every time. It assumes that those you care about may say one thing and do another; they may promise to stop a bad behavior but be guilty of recidivism. This is going to hurt you, but it won't devastate or paralyze you if you trust that you can deal with whatever happens.

We know we've said this before, but it bears repeating because it's so easy to forget: *You cannot control others.* However, you can trust people to behave according to their beliefs and historical patterns if they have not developed a new level of insight or made any personal growth. It's up to you to decide if you want to invest your trust while ignoring the past. You must also learn how to cope if the other person behaves contrary to his or her promise. Think about what you can trust yourself to do in adverse circumstances:

- ▶ You can trust yourself to quit a job when the boss promises you a promotion for the fourth time and fails to deliver.

- ▶ You can trust yourself to recognize that your child is going to continue to lie, cheat, and steal in order to obtain drugs and that he won't stop until you get him into a good treatment program.

- ▶ You can trust yourself to handle the disappointment and sadness when the person you've been dating decides to end the relationship, even though you had assumed that this was one that would last.

When you trust your own ability to deal with hurtful behavior and take action when you've reached your limit, then you're in a much better place psychologically to handle whatever is thrown at you. Rather than blindly trust other people to do what you think is right, you knowingly trust yourself to respond to them effectively.

Dealing With the Hurt: Options for Action

When you trust people to be themselves, you don't respond reflexively. You give yourself options. Too often, the parent whose child lies about his homework and the person whose spouse keeps cheating on her fall into familiar patterns. The parent says the same thing each time the child is caught in a lie, and the wife makes the same threats and exacts the same empty promises each time she catches her husband cheating. These patterns create tremendous anger and disappointment and nothing changes. If you trust people to be themselves, however, you moderate your own anger and disappointment. Rather than letting these powerful emotions govern your response, you provide yourself with other options. For example:

- ▶ You may choose to ignore the other person's behavior.
- ▶ You may choose to give the other person one more chance.

▶ You may choose to declare the behavior unacceptable.

▶ You may choose to forgive the other person.

The key is that it's your choice, based on your knowledge of how this person has behaved in the past and is likely to behave in the future.

In some instances, the evidence will convince you that you can trust people to be who they've made an effort to become. People can change to some degree—usually when it's too painful not to—and you may find that you believe absolutely that a particular person will stick to his or her new resolution or avoid certain behaviors. That's great. In other instances, however, you will need to choose to let go of the hurt and anger when someone acts according to his or her modus operandi. You are under no obligation, moral or otherwise, to restore someone to the role or place in your life he or she formerly occupied. Ending a friendship or marriage are options to be considered. You may need to take a "tough love" approach to your child and no longer demonstrate unconditional acceptance for everything he or she does. If you take these measures, remember that it does you no good to beat yourself up for what the other person does. Letting go of your negative feelings is crucial.

Remember, there are negotiables and non-negotiables. According to authors Basha Kaplan and Gail Prince, each person must know his or her own non-negotiables and set the bar or draw the line (Kaplan and Prince 1999). Using the four-step method discussed in Chapter 7 is helpful here because it allows you to set your personal expectations, share them with the other person, and assert your coping strategies and boundaries.

Steve, a therapist, had an office manager who embezzled money from his practice. When Steve discovered her dishonesty, he immediately asked for her key to the office and fired her. Steve was hurt and angry because she had stolen from him. Even though she had other minor criminal blemishes in the past, he was sure she was loyal to him. Still, he debated restoring her to her position of office manager. He was tempted to trust that she would learn from her lesson, and considered telling her about "dire consequences" if she ever did such a thing again. Ultimately, though, Steve realized he no longer trusted himself to feel safe and comfortable with this person. He would always be questioning what she was doing when she was in the office by herself; he would always wonder if his patients' information was safe. So he dismissed her. As much as Steve would have liked to give her another chance, he felt too vulnerable to do so. He trusted that she might return to her old behaviors. Some things are non-negotiable, and for Steve, having an honest office manager was one of them.

There is no foolproof way to know if you can trust someone not to make the same mistake again. If you do choose to forgive, recognize that the other person has the potential to disappoint you. At the same time, extend your trust without making your happiness contingent on his or her behavior. People who have unfaithful spouses sometimes want to forgive them, but then they say, "I don't want to risk being made a fool again." As the saying goes, it's not about you. The fool is the one who deceives, not the one who is deceived. Your kindly grandmother who falls for the insurance scam is not a fool; she trusted that the scam artist would do exactly what he said he would do. She is a person of her word, so she expected him to be also. That makes her vulnerable to deception, but this does not make her a fool. To choose to trust another does not imply naiveté or foolishness, but a choice to take another person at his or her word.

To take people at their word is a choice, a choice to trust not only in them but also in our ability to deal with the consequences of that choice. We may be hurt by our decision to trust someone, but we are not dumb, stupid, foolish, or any other negative quality because of what someone else does.

Here are some exercises that will facilitate trusting people to be themselves.

Exercises

Exercise 1—Identify a Trust Betrayed

With hindsight, it is easy to spot how we trust people to be who we want them to be, and then are hurt and disappointed when they act like themselves. Try this exercise to pinpoint one example of how this happened in your life.

1. Recall someone to whom you gave a second chance to behave the way you thought he or she should—a spouse, significant other, friend, child, boss, employee—and you were disappointed at what this person did with the chance. Write that person's name here:

    _____

2. Describe succinctly what past bad behavior you forgave (for example, cheating in a relationship or failing to meet deadlines for an employee):

    _____

    _____

    _____

3. Explain the second chance you gave to this person despite the negative behavior:

    _____

    _____

    _____

4. State what this person did with this second chance and how it made you feel:

    _____

    _____

    _____

5. Thinking back, describe why this person could have been expected to behave the way he/she did:

    _____

    _____

    _____

6. Describe what was going through your mind that allowed you to justify giving this person a second chance:

_____

_____

_____

Exercise 2—Trust Fantasies

Do you impose your own expectations on others? Here is an exercise that will allow you identify this tendency. Consider the following people in your life: spouse/significant other, sibling, parent, child, coworker, boss. Now, with each of these people in mind, answer the following questions:

▶ Do I often wish this person behaved differently than he or she usually does?

▶ Does this person often raise my hopes that he/she can change, and then act in ways that dash these hopes?

▶ Has our relationship fallen into a pattern in which I plead, threaten, or cajole in order to get this person to act differently, and then he/she manipulates me into believing that my actions are working?

▶ Does this person cause me significant emotional distress because I always trust that next time will be different (and next time isn't)?

Exercise 3—The Frankenstein Experiment

Choose the one person from the previous exercise who is most in need of a personality makeover. Imagine you have the power to turn this person into anyone you want him or her to be. Describe the new person you would create:

_____

_____

_____

_____

Now ask yourself the following questions:

▶ Is it feasible that the person you know could become this recreated person?

▶ Is it possible that he/she could at least acquire some of the traits of this "ideal"?

▶ Is it more realistic that he/she could change only in small ways in the direction you have sketched?

▶ Is it unlikely that this person can change in even the smallest way into the person you envisioned?

Chapter 10

Time Doesn't Heal All Pain; We Heal Ourselves By Learning to Let Go

Those who seek revenge should dig two graves.

—Chinese Proverb

Life is difficult.

—M. Scott Peck, *The Road Less Traveled*

One by one, the mourners paraded past the coffin to pay their respects. Kay listened to their kind words, including the suggestions that healing would come in time. Their advice was well-intentioned, but was it accurate? Do people heal emotionally simply due to the passage of time?

No, not exactly. Time heals nothing; it merely passes.

Yet if you're like most people, you probably believe that time has a curative power, and that each passing day dabs a little salve on an emotional wound. This belief is perfectly understandable, because most of us do feel a little better as we move further away in time from a traumatic event. What really is happening, though, is that time provides the opportunity for you to let go of your emotional pain. You feel better five years later because you have an opportunity to say good-bye to your loved one and shift your focus to other aspects of life, including the possibility of new relationships. Although you do feel better over time, it's a mistake to ascribe healing powers to the mere passing of weeks, months, or years. Doing so can foster the illusion that healing is a passive experience, that you don't have to do anything but sit there and let time work its magic. Unfortunately, it doesn't work this way. You probably know at least one person who is stuck in a grieving mode many years after a loss. To understand the value of this Truth, let's take a closer look at what happened to Kay after her loss.

How Kay Released Her Pain

Kay lost her only son, Mark, in a car accident when he had just turned 17. Time passed, but Kay continued to struggle with this loss. Suffering from depression, she showed up in therapy 20 years after the accident at the suggestion of her physician. During her first therapy session, she said that her husband of 30 years was dying, and the therapist assumed that this was the cause of her depression. In fact, Kay readily admitted that she and her husband were married only in the legal sense—the relationship had deteriorated years ago. His impending death was sad, but it wasn't sufficiently impactful to cause her depression. When he died, though, she started talking to her therapist about her son's death years ago.

Mark's death was so tragic and so unexpected, Kay didn't know what to do or how to survive after the accident. The daughter of an absent father and a controlling, demeaning mother, she felt her life had begun the moment her son was conceived. When he died, her life was extinguished with his. She celebrated his growth and development as the happiest part of her life. His accomplishments were proof positive of her worth; his disappointments were opportunities for her continued support in his life. When he died, she was bereft of hope, and the kind words offered by friends and family were meaningless. Her husband, too, provided no comfort. She felt him draw even further away, as if being close to her was a toxin that would kill him like it did their son. Her church friends were preachy, which wasn't helpful. Her mother was needy, a widow who wore her widowhood like a purple heart, but she was okay as long as Kay was there for her.

Kay finally made the decision to live. She didn't want to for her own sake, but there was no way she could desert her mother. That wouldn't be right. Kay took a job selling real estate. It would keep her busy during the day. She'd get more involved with mom—see her every day if that's what it took. If she were busy enough she wouldn't need to feel anything, and her various activities became coping strategies to avoid dealing with the emotional pain. Kay also took Valium for 20 years. She felt nothing thanks to the tranquilizer. In therapy, she asked, "What is it that I am supposed to feel?" Were it not for the Valium, Kay doubted that she would have survived. Nevertheless, there had been no healing. She needed to feel before she could heal. Kay didn't know how to feel anymore. Anything that reminded her of Mark, anything that prompted sadness or other painful emotions, was eliminated by Valium.

Ironically, her husband's death allowed her to start feeling again. It somehow jarred her sufficiently to recognize that her dependence on Valium was no longer enough to get her through. Her son had died a long time ago, and Kay may have understood that she had been paralyzed by grief for too long. She weaned herself off the drug. As a result, life was scarier. More than that, her anger broke through. She was angry with her father, with her late husband, with her dependent mother. She was even angry at God: "Where were you? How could you? How cruel can you be? If you truly knew the pain of losing your only son, how could you take mine?"

In one session, Kay talked to her therapist about a movie, *Turner and Hooch*, starring a young Tom Hanks. She watched it sorrowfully, never taking her eyes off the screen, with a pile of tissues accumulating in front of her. Mark looked just like Tom Hanks. It was as if he had come to life just to be in a silly story with a slobbering dog. It made her *feel*. She rented it again and watched it until she felt devoid of all tears and all emotion. Then she cried again. Having felt the pain of Mark's death, Kay grasped that he was gone for good. Intellectually, she had known this, of course. Emotionally, though, his death had finally sunk in and resonated with her. She was able to say good-bye to him in a way she had never done before.

She expressed her feelings in letters she wrote to the dead: Mark, her father, her husband. She even wrote to God, cursing him at first but then softening and confessing her heart was broken. She opened her Bible and read as she wept quietly. Beneath her rage, Kay uncovered the sadness that was her most powerful link to Mark. The pain, which she had kept frozen inside her for the last 20 years since Mark's death, was free at last. And Kay was free—to feel, to express, to let go.

In releasing the pain, Kay was releasing Mark; she could feel that. She was also releasing herself from the burden that she had carried for so long, the burden of living an emotionless life—a life devoid of joy and sorrow, belly laughs and deep sadness—a life of slow, torturous survival. In giving herself permission to say good-bye to Mark, Kay was again allowing herself to experience life in its raw form. She was returning to the place of being a fully feeling and functioning human being. By learning to let go of her pain, Kay changed from a broken, robotic human being to a happy, grateful woman. For the first time in her life, she was able to set boundaries with her needy, controlling mother, and in so doing, became much more intimate with and less resentful of her. Kay also fell in love with a widower, and they had the type of relationship she had always dreamed about when she was younger.

Kay healed herself. She was actively involved in the process of letting go of Mark. Rather than passively wait for time to dull the hurt, Kay did the grieving work necessary, both with her therapist and outside of therapy, to let go fully. This was the key to her emotional healing.

We want to emphasize that this Truth is about all types of healing and not just about recovering from the death of a loved one. Many times we incur serious emotional pain and become stuck in some counterproductive attitude or behavior. We are fired from a job we love and are so bitter and resentful that we can't function effectively in any job. We are betrayed by someone we love and become mired in distrust, unable to find another partner or sustain a meaningful relationship. As with the death of a loved one, we are passive in the face of this pain, trusting that time will help us get past whatever emotion or situation that has us in its grip. What we should be doing, though, is learning to let go. Let's look at how you can learn the critical five steps of the process.

Five Steps to Emotional Healing

As you can see from Kay's story, healing can be a complicated process for a variety of reasons. You may trust that time will heal your wounds and waste months or years waiting for it to happen. You may be stuck in a state of shame or guilt with no appreciation for what it takes to heal. It's likely that you're not aware of the five steps that are required to heal. Each step is necessary, as it is difficult to recover and reach an emotionally healthy place without each of them. The first three steps prepare you for releasing the pain, and the fourth step involves the actual letting go. Here are the five steps, followed by a discussion of each:

1. Remembering.
2. Feeling.
3. Expressing.
4. Releasing.
5. Changing your thinking.

Remembering

We must return to the part of our life that created the wound. Going around it or blocking it from the conscious mind does not promote healing. The mind has the capacity to occlude painful and unacceptable memories and feelings for decades to aid in its survival. A relevant metaphor is that of a teapot. When you turn the flame on, the water gradually heats. When it reaches the boiling point, steam flows out of the spout. If the spout is clogged or blocked, however, the steam builds up. Over time, the pressure becomes great enough to crack the teapot. When we fail to remember, we are like the broken teapot. When we wall off key memories and feelings and don't experience them fully (or at all), an essential part of ourselves breaks. Like Kay, we may be aware of the traumatic event in our past and make a conscious effort to keep it isolated. This can also be an unconscious process, in which we don't realize what events and feelings we're avoiding. In both instances, this failure of memory harms our emotional well-being.

Unconscious blockage of critical memories is especially insidious. In psychological terms, this is called *repression* or *motivated forgetting*. The University of Oregon's Dr. Michael Anderson is an expert in this area. He suggests that our unremembered, compartmentalized material is only ready to be processed years later, when we are prepared to know, accept, and release the reality of what we experienced earlier in our lives (*Newsweek*, March 27, 2006). Gina, for instance, is now in her mid-70s but only recently acknowledged the sexual molestation she experienced during her childhood years. The shame that she felt, the recurrent dreams of being chased, and the inability to walk away from a horrible marriage all testify to the power that her abuser has wielded over her for decades. To heal, Gina must remember and return to the experience that created the emotional pain. That is, she must be willing to talk about a part of her life that she has never spoken to anyone about until recently. But how?

The key is finding a listener whom you trust implicitly. Many times, this person is a therapist. When you trust this person as well as the process by which you reveal an emotionally painful event, you feel safer to articulate the truth than you would in other circumstances. A therapist can provide a sense of security and caring and a belief in you. "Take me to the pain" is an instruction we frequently provide. In response to the therapist, the client takes the initiative and leads the therapist to the wound. For complete healing to occur, all of the contents of the traumatic memory box must be emptied. In fact, some patients return to a painful experience or trauma a second or third time because they hadn't fully remembered or articulated all their painful experiences. Only by addressing these experiences in their totality can you put yourself on the road to letting them go.

Feeling

It is not enough to remember or even verbalize a painful event. The event must be felt. In many instances, it has never been felt. If that sounds like a surprising statement, consider that Kay never felt Mark's death because of her use of Valium and other protective strategies. This is also where you will most likely become stuck in the healing process. As psychologist Dr. Renee Fredrickson has said in her lectures, "It's about the feelings." People avoid thinking about the traumas of their past not because of the experience itself, but because of the emotional hurt. It is the fear experienced during a drunken father's rage that they never want to feel again. It may be the helplessness that engulfed them during a terrible car crash that they avoid remembering. Or it can involve the shame they experienced as a child when their parents divorced.

Many times patients resist entering these feeling states because of the extreme pain involved, but the obstacle is not so much re-experiencing the pain as it is feeling it for the first time. People frequently experience the trauma and leave the pain there. For example, a frightened child may remove herself mentally and emotionally from a traumatic scene (a concept known as *dissociation*) and watch it from a removed vantage point. Consequently, the feelings are never processed, and the reality is never fully experienced. Although this protects the child temporarily, she can't completely heal from the experience because she can't express and release what she never felt in the first place. Years later, often in the safety of a therapist's office, she may finally allow the trauma to enter her consciousness enough to feel, express, and release the emotion she has avoided for most of her life.

Unfinished feelings (also called *unresolved feelings*) are emotions that have never been processed. A therapist might say to you, "It sounds as if you have never dealt with your mother's death" or "You seem to have unresolved anger surrounding your divorce." What this means is that these events and the feelings associated with them still have power in your life. No doubt, some of you may feel like you're tough enough to handle these unresolved feelings—that you can keep them locked away so they don't hurt you or anyone else. In fact, no one is "tough enough." Why would you want to keep this terrible pain to yourself anyway? More to the point, carrying it around inside of you for years impacts you in negative ways that you might be unaware of.

Scott is a small-college basketball coach with a passion for winning. His passion is not only about amassing victories for his personal resume but also about his players. In fact, he is so protective of these players that his athletic director at the college ordered him to see a therapist for anger management counseling. On more than one occasion, he's confronted opposing coaches after hard fouls on his players and threatened these coaches with bodily harm if such fouls reoccurred. Although Scott was genuinely concerned for his players, he communicates that concern in a rage. He seems completely out of control as he threatens the coaches from other teams. Scott understood that he was overreacting in these situations but didn't understand why he behaved the way he did. When his therapist asked him to identify the source of the fear that culminated in such a strong need to protect his players, Scott said, "It's not fear, man. It's anger!"

"Okay," the therapist agreed, "then tell me about the anger."

Scott eventually told the therapist that as a boy, he watched his father beat his mother mercilessly while he stood frozen with helplessness and terror. *Never again*, he thought. No one would ever hurt anyone Scott loved while he passively stood by. Scott had walled off the feelings from this memory, if not the memory itself. This may seem like a minor distinction, but it was anything but minor for Scott. Resisting the intense and terrifying feelings protected Scott from the pain of his childhood, but it mutated into counterproductive behaviors in his adult years. By expressing his feelings about what happened, Scott was able to differentiate between the past and the present. In other words, the fouls that his players sustained were not the same as the physical beatings his mother endured. Thus, Scott saw how the angry threats he directed at other coaches were an overreaction to the current situation and no longer a viable option. He removed permission to behave in such a manner and worked on new ways to think about these situations, formulating a plan to behave in a more appropriate manner during games.

Expressing

As important as it was that Scott felt his feelings, he needed to do more. Thinking about what happened when he was a boy and feeling the anger and fear he experienced then were simply the first two steps on the path to letting go of his pain. As Scott discovered, he needed to express his feelings as part of this process. These kinds of feelings may be expressed in spoken or written words and are often accompanied by tears. They may be expressed to an individual (a sponsor, a therapist, a loved one) or a group (a circle of friends or a support group).

Melanie's physician referred her to a therapist after he could find no neurological basis for a sudden seizure, suspecting that the seizure was anxiety-induced. Melanie was stressed out by her family, and she admitted that she had become a bitter woman who resented every family member. Her brother had sexually molested her. Her father abandoned the family and then died young. Her mother never protected her from her brother's advances, nor did she believe her when Melanie told her about the abuse. Her own husband had failed her in countless ways.

Borrowing some tools and techniques from psychologist Dr. Syd Simon, the therapist challenged Melanie to complete a multi-part assignment for each of her family members. The first task was to write him/her a letter describing from Melanie's perspective: 1) what happened, 2) how it felt to be her at the time, 3) how it has affected her since, and 4) what she will do now to let it go. (Many people do an excellent job of steps 1 through 3 because they are very angry with the person who hurt them. Step 4 is more difficult because it requires the letter writer to assume the responsibility of letting go of the pain, the fourth step in the process.) The therapist then gave Melanie a second and even more challenging task: Write a letter from each family member's perspective *as if she were that person*, telling herself what she needed to hear to help release the pain. For example:

> Dear Melanie,
>
> It has taken me years to write this letter to you. I've never
> wanted to confront the reality of what I did to you as a child.

Third, the therapist asked Melanie to compose a list of 10 events or circumstances from the life of the particular family member in question that "made him/her the person they became." Why the third exercise? To help Melanie understand that the other person's behavior is about him or her, and that Melanie should not take responsibility and ownership for that person's unique history. When Melanie focused on her father and why he abandoned her, she determined that his own father abandoned their family when he was 3 years old; she also noted that his mother was very critical and controlling of him. Melanie added that her father didn't have the skills or courage to parent four kids.

All three of these exercises helped Melanie express feelings that had been bottled inside her for years. Some of them were difficult for her; her conversations with her therapist were often punctuated by tears. After having gone through this process, however, Melanie reported that her resentment had dissipated, and was replaced by a sense of relief and peace. As difficult as it was to express her feelings and talk about extremely painful experiences from her past, it was cathartic. Not only did she feel better about herself and her life after this expression, but she never experienced another seizure.

Releasing

Letting go of emotional hurt follows its expression, but it is not always synonymous with its expression. In other words, some people may cling to their painful experiences despite talking about them. Interestingly, when people cry, it's often a sign that they're moving toward letting go. It suggests that an individual has reached the core of the emotional wound. Spilling the hurt into a tissue is often exactly what the doctor ordered. But to let go of a toxic emotion fully and permanently, people need to move beyond tears and forgive.

We all know of people who cry themselves to sleep over the same issue night after painful night. If they are feeling their feelings and expressing them, why are they not healing? Some people hold on to their feelings despite expressing them. Though they may not know why they're doing this, they hold on to toxic emotions for a variety of reasons—to keep a departed person "alive," to avoid the responsibility that comes with happiness and success, to protect themselves from the scariness of loving someone, and so on. Forgiveness and letting go diminishes our desire to hold on to these emotions. When we forgive, we're not condoning, excusing, or minimizing the bad things that someone else may have done. Nor is it about evening the score or being weak. We forgive others from a position of strength— the strength to release pain and anger without calling for vengeance or demanding an apology from the offender.

Research suggests that people are much more inclined to forgive another person if they receive an apology, even if the apology is insincere. Be aware, however, that the people in your past not only may not apologize, they may deny they ever committed the act that scarred you in the first place. We've had a number of patients through the years who have experienced remarkable personal growth and found the courage to confront family members about past abuse. Unfortunately, the other family members have not experienced any personal growth or change and don't acknowledge what they did or are in denial about their contributions to the problem. Consequently, the person who complains of the abuse is invalidated and sometimes ostracized from the family who rallies to the defense of the accused.

Although forgiveness is easier when validation and apology exist, they are not necessary. People who were abused as children can learn to let go of this emotional pain as adults, even when the abusers have died a long time ago. These abusers can't apologize or admit guilt, yet these victims of abuse are able to forgive. They understand a corollary to this chapter's Truth: Forgiveness is a gift we give to ourselves, not necessarily to the person who did us wrong. Forgiveness is one (though not the only) method available to let go of a hurt that has bothered and limited us for years. Consider the research that suggests that forgiving benefits the forgiver medically and psychologically. The person who learns to forgive is significantly less likely to suffer a fatal heart attack, strokes, depression, and anxiety disorders than the resentful person. We don't pretend to grasp the medical reasons why this is so, but from a psychological perspective, we can speculate that forgiveness is a way of taking the deep hurt we have suffered and saying that, despite how awful an experience might have been, we can now release it. It is liberating to forgive—it fills us with peace rather than feelings of hate, resentment, fear, and shame.

Letting go doesn't always involve forgiving someone, however. Sometimes it simply means saying good-bye. Given today's longer life expectancy, we can expect multiple losses to contend with, from friends to family members. Sometimes letting go means accepting the loss of a valued relationship, as Martha was able to do. Martha carried a deep wound for almost 25 years as the result of a skirmish with her daughter. She felt a sense of bitter betrayal from a choice her daughter made to exclude her from a family function. Her hurt was not healed by the passing of a quarter of a century. If anything, the hurt was stronger years later than it was right after the incident occurred. As our Truth indicates, time itself does not heal; it only passes.

Martha was a willing participant in therapy. She quickly discovered that she was reinforcing her bitterness and strengthening her hurt because she could not let go of her negative feelings. Her therapist explained that her daughter did what she did because it made sense to her at the time— from her perspective, at that instant, it made sense to her daughter to exclude Martha. She could hold on to it for more years and stew over it, or she could let it go. She could reconcile with her daughter or not, but she no longer needed to keep the pain fresh by reliving the hurtful exclusion again and again. (Martha kept replaying the incident in her head and telling herself how she had been terribly wronged.)

Once Martha understood that she had a choice, she decided it was time to let go of the pain. This required an action, not just a mental commitment to letting go. She wrote her daughter a letter (one she did not send) to express her feelings and to say a final good-bye to her hurt and resentment. The result was almost magical to Martha; she released her pain and anger in one session after feeding it for 25 years. She elected to make peace with the fact that she had positive relationships with many other family members, including her two other children. Martha realized that the relationship with her daughter may have been irreparably damaged, but at least she would no longer suffer from her bitterness and hurt.

By letting go and healing, Martha put herself in a position to love and be hurt again. Like most people who don't let go, Martha had created a protective barrier designed to keep herself from feeling both love and hurt. She allowed herself to feel emotions such as resentment and bitterness, but she also cut herself off from loving and the vulnerability that accompanies caring for another. In a sense, Martha was living in an emotionally cool place where the warmer emotions couldn't penetrate. This meant no great joy and no great hurt, but that was not an emotionally healthy way to live.

Perhaps you understand Martha's need to protect herself from strong emotion. By not letting go of that initial hurt, she provided herself with a reminder not to get too close to other people, because they might hurt in the way that her daughter had. Many people in therapy hold on to resentment, and blame their present problems on a series of negative events from the past. Though the events might have been painful and tragic, the patients attempt to control and blame others for problems that they should own, especially if they intend to heal. Staying stuck in blaming others absolves an individual of responsibility for cleaning up the messes they have made in life. Despite the trauma suffered, people who choose to continue in their unhealthy patterns of behavior are no longer victims of these behaviors—they are volunteers.

Why would anyone volunteer to hold onto emotional wounds? Because (as you'll see the following parable), doing so provides an anesthetic for the pain, even as it numbs us to all the positive feelings we might experience. Consider the analogy provided in Henry's story. Henry was walking home late one winter evening on a cold Pennsylvania night. Henry was not wearing gloves and kept his hands nestled in his pockets for protection from the sub-freezing temperature. As he walked, Henry failed to notice a patch of ice that launched him into a less-than-acrobatic, face-first dive onto the pavement. The blow registered neurologically in the region of the brain that governs the olfactory nerve, which governs the sense of smell. For an extended time, Henry lost his ability to smell anything. He perceived this as a blessing initially, because he could walk past garbage dumps or open sewers and not smell their foul odors. Soon, however, he noticed a downside to his injury. On a camping trip with the guys, he became acutely aware of the evergreen trees and the wonderful aroma he could no longer enjoy. The once intoxicating smell of the campfire was lost to Henry. Gone also were camping's familiar morning enticements of coffee and bacon.

Think about how Henry's quality of life was diminished by losing his sense of smell. Now think about how our quality of life is diminished when we lose our capacity to experience emotion fully. When we don't release our hurt, we gradually become numb to situations and events until we lose all contact with our emotional selves. To help you release your emotional pain effectively, we've compiled a list of effective tools as follows:

Artistic expression

We already noted how Melanie used writing as a way to release toxic emotions. Other art forms are equally effective. For centuries, poetry has been a popular form of expressing hurt. Emotional pain can also be released through drawing, sculpture, and painting. Some people prefer to express themselves in music or dance. As Elton John wrote, "Sad songs mean so much." And consider Gloria Gaynor's passionate "I will survive!"

You don't need to be a professional artist to take advantage of these modes of expression; you don't even need to be particularly talented. John, 17, talked with his therapist about the pain he had been nurturing throughout his adolescence because his father abandoned him to live with another family in a distant place, and John rarely saw him. Once he expressed his pain, John worked on releasing his feelings and making peace with his loss. When the therapist suggested John use the letter-writing technique described earlier, he declined, saying, "No, I know what I need to do." What he did was go into the woods and bang on his bongos until he had expressed and released the anguish he felt from his father's disappearance.

Prayer

In one of her lectures to the Florida Psychological Association, Dr. Ruben asserted that "happiness begins with a daily prayer." She, like millions of others, believes that prayer is another way to release emotional pain. Many religions espouse the belief that a higher power is capable of removing unwanted feelings, not to mention impulses, "sins," and self-defeating thoughts. From a psychological perspective, belief governs emotions. To believe that God, Allah, Jehovah, Jesus, Zeus, or a shaman can alleviate your emotional pain may ensure that the pain will dissipate. People of faith have shared countless anecdotal accounts of their faith's power to restore them to wholeness after a devastating loss. Is this healing based solely on belief or is there something more supernatural involved in healing emotional pain? This is likely more of a matter of opinion and faith and less of a matter of science. Or is it? In the book *Healing Words*, physician Larry Dossey cites compelling research that prayer is a scientifically valid approach to healing emotional and physical ailments. He concludes that prayer complements the practice of "good medicine."

Sublimation

In 1980, Candi Lightner created Mothers Against Drunk Driving (M.A.D.D.) in Sacramento, California, after her 13-year-old daughter, Cari, was killed by a drunk driver. Her anguish at losing a child devastated and incapacitated Ms. Lightner, but she didn't give up and withdraw from life. Instead, she reinvested her pain in a cause she was passionate about. Her ability to exchange a self-destructive rage for the opportunity to save lives illustrates the Freudian concept of *sublimation*, which is the reinvestment of unconscious sexual energy in other passionate pursuits. Many mental health professionals since Freud have widened the definition to include other emotional energies, as well. It's a way of taking painful feelings such as fear, guilt, sadness, and anxiety and reinvesting them by doing something positive with that same emotional energy. In this way, emotional hurt is released by transforming it into a passionate pursuit.

Guided imagery

In guided imagery, therapists help their patients imagine people, scenarios or conversations. The way it works is simple: People close their eyes and envision themselves accomplishing something that is otherwise impossible in reality. For example, you confront an abuser who has long been deceased, you say good-bye to a family member who passed away decades ago, or you express mixed feelings to those who have died prematurely. Guided imagery can also help you resolve the unresolved, such as a devastating car accident or a combat-related trauma. From the therapist's perspective, it is a tool to help patients look at a painful scene from a different perspective, from that of a survivor rather than a victim. People can finally say good-bye to someone or something that has tortured them for years.

Why is guided imagery such an effective technique? In a sense, it's a trick, because perception is reality. Our nervous system does not know the difference between reality and imagination. If our minds see something happen, our bodies process it as real. That is why dreams are so powerful. The accompanying emotions are often as powerful as if the dream really had happened. In the same way, guided imagery creates a powerful sense of emotional reality—it helps people let go of emotional hurt in the same way as the other techniques discussed. (One caveat: We do not recommend using it without the assistance of a trained professional, especially if you are attempting to resolve a long-standing trauma or abusive scene.)

Changing your thinking

This fifth and final step provides a cognitive compliment to the affective work patients do. As you recall from our first Truth, thinking impacts feeling. You must think well to feel well. Our experiences as therapists as well as the literature in our field provide ample evidence that positive thinking is enormously helpful in the healing process, if not curative in and of itself. King Solomon wrote in the Old Testament book of Proverbs (17:22): "A merry heart does good like a medicine." Norman Vincent Peale in his classic work described the magical powers of positive thinking. More recently, Dr. Martin Seligman developed a system of thought called Positive Psychotherapy (PPT), outlined in his book *Authentic Happiness*. It rests on the belief that depression can be helped by building positive emotions through changing thoughts, attitudes, and beliefs.

Lou was involved in a car accident with multiple fatalities. He walked away physically unscathed. The accident was not his fault, but he was haunted by the experience. Treatment required flushing out the specifics of what happened and, most importantly, what bothered him. Then he had to feel, express, and release his emotions to gain peace. Healing also required him to think differently about the accident, as he was suffering from survivor's guilt. He had to replace unhealthy cognitions such as "I have no right to be happy if those people are dead" and "I can never feel safe on the road again" with more rational thoughts such as "The accident was not my fault. I cannot bring the victims back to life by torturing myself" and "I have been driving safely for more than 50 years. I can return to the road a confident, cautious driver once again."

To change your thinking, you need to change your life plan. This means not only saying good-bye to the loss, but also saying hello to what is next. To learn and grow, you must master the art of replacement, detaching from that which is gone and reattaching to that which is here. When you can no longer play, you coach. Your dog died? There is an adorable homeless puppy waiting for you at the Humane Society. Your favorite program is off the air? Find a new one. Lose another job? Get off that couch and pound the pavement!

It's also possible to change your plan regarding people. This may not involve a simple replacement—a live dog for a dead one—but the principle applies. Most mental health professionals agree that jumping from one relationship to another without a grieving period is unhealthy. An opportunity to say good-bye to the loved one, to feel and experience that loss and learn something about the self—these actions are healthy. When those tasks have been successfully completed, however, opening ourselves to love again is a way of reinvesting after loss. Risking intimacy always means risking loss (and the accompanying sadness), but it reflects a decision to start living life again, albeit with an altered plan.

Dave was a firemedic (firefighter and paramedic) who retired to another state on disability. He sought the services of a psychologist to address symptoms of posttraumatic stress disorder. One symptom involved a recurring nightmare: Dave would awaken with the memory of being chased down a boulevard by an assortment of human body parts that he had found detached from accident survivors at one point or another throughout his extended career. Dave had not dealt with or "finished" these incidents by appropriately grieving them. That is, he needed to tell his stories and express and release his feelings about what had happened. Dave needed to share with someone what it felt like to arrive at the scene of an accident and save a young man with a severed arm. He had reached a time in his life when it was necessary to take the memories of incidents like this out of mental storage and tell them to someone who could help him make sense of his reactions and feelings. By doing so, Dave could release the feelings and eliminate the nightmares.

Note that his healing encapsulated all the steps of the process: remembering (returning to the incident); experiencing his feelings (a luxury a firemedic does not have at the time of the incident); expressing his feelings; releasing his feelings; and, finally, thinking differently about the incidents. Note that steps one through four occurred almost seamlessly; he shared and released his memories and feelings in the telling of each of his stories. The fifth step, thinking differently, embraced new concepts: "I did the best I could for each survivor. I made a difference in many lives. I cannot change what I cannot control."

This five-step theory is one of several that exist. The works of Robert Ackerman, Susan Forward, and Dr. Syd Simon explore others. There are also models on the process of forgiveness, including Enright and Fitzgibbons (2000) and a more recent expansion of that model incorporating feminist principles (McKay et. al., 2007). Whatever model you choose, however, recognize that you need to take charge of your healing instead of trusting in time to heal you. As you go through life, you will experience emotional pain, whether in the form of loss, betrayal, abandonment, rejection, abuse, or, most commonly, all of these. In order to live life free of apathy, resentment, addiction/compulsions, emotional numbing, and a hardening of the spirit, you need to learn how to let go. To be a healthy human being requires the capacity to release pain. It is to love, to lose, to hurt, to say good-bye, to heal, and then to do it all again. The cycle is repeated thousands of times in a lifetime with people, events, and dreams.

Now let's explore how these five steps for emotional healing can work for you in the following exercises.

Exercises

Exercise 1—Dr. Syd Simon's Expression Exercise

To express your feelings, take the following three actions:

1. Write a letter to the person responsible for your emotional wound (but don't show or send it to the person), specifying what happened, how you felt at the time, how it has affected you since, and what you're going to do now to let go of your negative feeling.

2. Write a letter from the perspective of the person who caused you this pain, telling you what you need to know so you can release it.

3. Compose a list of 10 events that caused this person to become the person he/she is.

Exercise 2—Sublimation

The goal of this exercise is to help you identify how you might redirect your emotional energy in a positive direction. Answer the following questions to determine the cause that you might best serve, and that might also serve you.

1. What social issue concerns you the most? What issue do you think and talk about the most?

2. Is there a volunteer group addressing this cause in your community where you might devote a certain amount of time weekly?

If you're having difficulty finding the right group or cause, do the following:

1. Make a list of five problems in the world you're most concerned about (illiteracy, global warming, and so on).

2. Go on the Internet and do a search using the name of each issue and your city or geographical area.

3. Create a list of five possible local volunteer organizations based on your search, one for each problem.

4. Prioritize the list in terms of what you've read online about each group and the types of volunteers they need. Then call the top priority and volunteer.

Exercise 3—Guided Imagery

Find a quiet location. Find a comfortable position, either sitting or lying down. If you find that you need to sleep during this process, please do not fight the urge as this will cause more stress. If you are distracted, do not fight the external stimulus. Take note of the distraction and then return to the exercise. Focus on your breathing. Expand your abdominal cavity by taking deep breaths. Hold for one count longer than you normally would and then release. Practice makes this process easier. Consider the situation, problem, or event at hand. Now imagine it in a different light. See yourself handling it differently, more constructively. Observe others' behavior as a reflection of them. Your reactions are statements about yourself. Now, think positive and constructive thoughts to lead you to optimal outcomes.

Exercise 4—Practice Changing Your Thoughts

To help you shift your thinking in ways that release painful emotions, practice rethinking. Let's start out with a relatively easy scenario: You forget to pick up your spouse's favorite cookies at the store, and she's mad at you. In response, you think: "I am stupid and inconsiderate; she'll probably divorce me before the year ends, and I deserve to be divorced." Now rethink that thought and write three possible positive alternatives. For instance: "I'm human and made a mistake. Most of the time I'm thoughtful, and I'll be sure not to forget the next time she asks me to do something."

_____

_____

_____

_____

_____

_____

Try to apply this rethinking to an emotionally difficult situation in your life, one in which you beat yourself up because of how events transpired. Maybe it was a divorce. Maybe it's estrangement from a sibling or parent. In the following space, write the original, negative thought that keeps running through your mind, then rewrite the thought in a positive manner:

_____

_____

_____

_____

_____

_____

_____

Chapter 11

Putting the 10 Truths to Work for You

At this point, you may be working hard to process the 10 Truths and thinking about how to integrate them into your life. There is plenty to think about, and you may find yourself wondering how you can put all these principles into practice. That last word is key. Practice. If you keep a list of the Truths handy and look at them occasionally, they'll gradually become part of your consciousness. You'll naturally become more aware of how these psychological principles apply to your life. After a while, each Truth will become part of how you think about and deal with life situations. For instance, when you wonder why you are dating someone you know isn't good for you, you'll realize you've given yourself permission to date guys who are charming rogues but will end up hurting you. If you're wise and decide to apply this Truth to your life, you won't give yourself permission to date this type of person.

We're making this sound easier than it actually is. Most people don't go from dating guys who are bad for them to dating ones who are good for them overnight. That's where practice comes in. You need to practice not only thinking about these Truths but also trying them out in various situations. After a while, you'll internalize the Truths, and using them to deal with a variety of issues will become second nature. To help you with this internalization process, we're going to provide you with a *practicum*— ways to practice what you've learned within the controlled environment of this book. We're going to take you through three different scenarios in order for you to gain proficiency in applying the Truths. Unlike previous chapters where we've inserted exercises at the end, these are integrated into the chapter itself. In medical school, the mantra is "see one, do one, teach one," but we're offering a slight variation on this. The first part of the chapter asks you to "see" and think about a case history involving Edward; the second part requires you to "do" (apply) the Truths after reading about Laurie; and the third part is about "teaching"—turning the Truths on yourself and personalizing the lessons learned.

A Challenging Case: Analyzing How the Truths Apply

Edward is a 42-year-old history teacher married to an English teacher, and they have one child, a 7-year-old girl. Edward can't stop obsessing about the unlikely possibility that his wife is having an extra-marital relationship with a 19-year-old employee at the school where they both work. What makes the problem embarrassing for Edward is that he has stooped to violating his wife's personal boundaries by reading her e-mails and checking her cell phone records. He has found nothing incriminating. He knows his spying is wrong. In fact, he knows the affair is not happening, but he can't stop himself from worrying about it. As a result, he is driving himself and his wife crazy with his incessant questions. These questions have become unfounded accusations, further endangering their marriage.

Edward was an only child, and he had a close relationship with his mother and a pleasant, if not close, relationship with his father. He was a good student with several school friends, although he was not popular and never a ladies' man. He did, however, have a relationship with a woman when he was 22 that ended badly when she started sleeping with a friend of his. Growing up, Edward was not involved in conflicts with anyone and described himself as having a moderate amount of social self-confidence and above average academic self-confidence. When Edward was 14, his mother left his father. She invited her son to join her, but Edward could not leave his father, feeling his father would then be completely alone. Edward did well in college, and he met his wife who was also an education major. They married three months after graduation and both landed jobs in the same middle school. A few years later, they had their daughter, and Edward was fine at this point.

After his daughter was born, however, Edward became obsessive about two things. The first time he became consumed with worry when his daughter was diagnosed with a severe case of chicken pox. Although she was very ill, she fortunately recovered completely. The second time was when his doctor told him he had a brain tumor. Again, fortunately, it turned out not to be life-threatening—the doctors determined it was benign. In both cases, Edward had agonized over potentially fatal situations, both of which amounted to little more than false alarms.

Now let's examine how the Truths helped Edward deal with the issues in his life.

Truth #1: Emotions are not mysterious visitors; they can be identified and understood.

This Truth allowed Edward to recognize that his feelings made sense to him. In other words, he saw that his anxiety was not a byproduct of his situation, his wife's behavior, or that of her 19-year-old acquaintance. Instead, it was his perception of the relationship between his wife and the young man that caused his emotions. He sensed a threat where there was no evidence of misdeed. As Edward thought about it, he realized that the combination of his love for his wife and what appeared to be suspicious circumstances spiked his anxiety. Once Edward was able to admit that his anxiety was about him rather than the innocent situation or the other people, his anxiety no longer seemed strange and scary. He could see how it arose from who he was and how he perceived things.

Truth #2: You can change your compulsive behaviors if you change your thoughts and address your feelings.

Using this second Truth, Edward became aware that his compulsive behavior—his spying and checking up on his wife—could be changed if he altered his thoughts and feelings. He realized how this compulsive behavior had a purpose—it protected him from vulnerability and gave him a sense of control over the situation between his wife and her young acquaintance. The worry took on a life of its own and persisted despite some very real consequences for Edward and his wife. Recognizing that he needed to change how he thought and felt if he wanted to manage his compulsion, Edward explored different methods to do so: biochemically, through the sensorimotor system, and cognitively. Edward did not want to take medication, and he wasn't particularly interested in using exercise to change his feelings. Instead, Edward chose to express his feelings to his therapist, resulting in a sense of what Edward termed "relief."

Truth #3: Every behavior has an underlying purpose, and it's not always what we think.

Edward used this Truth to recognize that his compulsion had an underlying motivation. The more Edward reflected on why he engaged in his self-defeating behavior, the clearer he became as to its origin. Edward had had two previous episodes in which he was controlled by excessive worry, one concerning his daughter's health and the other, his own health. Both times the problems disappeared without serious consequences. In fact, he admitted that the worry seemed to bring about the desired outcome. When he realized that his anxiety was magical thinking, he saw how he used it as a kind of talisman against catastrophe.

Truth #4: We all sabotage ourselves unless we confront our internal saboteur.

Edward hired his saboteur to protect him from the fear of loss, especially of important relationships. Edward's epiphany was that he had become very sensitive to and fearful of abandonment ever since his mother left when he was a teenager and after his girlfriend's infidelity when he was 22. He feared his daughter would abandon him through death, and his wife would abandon him through infidelity. His fear was powerful although not consciously understood. He avoided dealing directly with his fear by creating a self-sabotaging worry machine that tortured him and his wife.

Truth #5: All behavior requires permission so we must learn what we're permitting ourselves to do.

Edward permitted himself to respond to his life situations in several ways. He would not let himself abandon his father when his mother left. He did not let himself reestablish a close relationship with his mother.

They still had a relationship, but Edward kept her at arm's length. He would not permit himself to forgive his mother for leaving. Consequently, Edward did not allow himself to trust anyone else to love him and stay with him. Instead, he allowed himself to worry obsessively, interrogate his wife, and snoop behind her back. When Edward became aware of what his permissions involved, he was embarrassed. He realized he was permitting himself to say and do things that he found unacceptable.

Truth #6: Emotional energy is finite and needs to be invested rather than wasted on wishing, worrying, and whining.

Edward was wasting his emotional energy on imagining romantic encounters between his wife and her school acquaintance. This Truth shifted Edward's perspective. Though he came to understand that he was worrying unnecessarily, the concept of wasting emotional energy really hit home. He was keenly aware of how enervating his incessant agonizing was, leaving him little emotional energy for anything else in his life.

Truth #7: Our relationships depend on self-empowerment and not on enabling others.

It dawned on Edward that he was attempting to control his wife, and that by spying on her, he was diminishing his own power and making his greatest fear the single most powerful thing in his life. From this Truth, Edward realized he needed to shift from enabling others to self-empowerment, and he did it using the four steps we discussed in Chapter 7. Here's how Edward translated these steps in a self-empowerment exercise:

> Step 1—Express feelings appropriately. "I am frightened of the possibility of losing you because I realize how important you are to me. I love you and have invested more in this relationship than any other in my life. I want to stay with you until death do us part, as we said in our marriage vows."

> Step 2—Make a specific request. "Please be faithful to me as I will be to you."

Step 3—Set boundaries for yourself. "I choose not to attempt to control you, question you, or spy on you any more, but I will not stay in a relationship with infidelity. I will leave if you choose to be unfaithful."

Step 4—Take proper care of yourself. "I know I can't control you so I will take care of me. I will respond appropriately if the time comes when you demonstrate that you choose not to be faithful to me."

We should note that the statements Edward made as part of the previous four steps were ones directed at himself; he didn't share them with others, nor did he need to for them to be effective in his healing.

Truth #8: Ego boundaries protect us from rejection, insult, and intimidation.

This Truth provided Edward with insight into why he had been so hurt by his mother's and his girlfriend's behavior, and his own need to draw lines that protected him from the actions of others. He came to see that his mother's decision to leave his father was all about her need to get away from her husband, not to hurt him. He also recognized that that his girlfriend who cheated on him years earlier needed excessive external validation and attention. Her behavior was a reflection of her own values and not a statement about him. Most significantly, Edward grasped that he needed to set boundaries to protect himself from what others might do or what he imagined they were doing. If his wife were to be unfaithful, this behavior would reflect on her, not on him. This conferred an internal sense of security on Edward, making him less easily disturbed by his fantasies about what his wife might be doing.

Truth #9: You can trust people to be who they are, not who you want them to be.

In a way, this was Edward's most crucial Truth. He realized that he could choose to trust that his wife would be faithful to him—she was a loyal, caring person, and this trait made it highly unlikely that she would act in ways that his imagination had conjured. More powerfully, he decided to trust himself to respond to the situation with grace and dignity, regardless of her decisions and behavior. Edward placed his trust in God, his wife, and himself—instead of the magical power of his worries—to reinstate the peace of mind he had forfeited after learning about his wife's school acquaintance. He understood that his fears were not well-founded but had their origins in how his mother and girlfriend had acted many years ago.

Truth #10: Time doesn't heal all pain; we heal ourselves by learning how to let go.

Edward learned that he was holding on to things that prevented peace of mind and healing. First, he was keeping resentment, especially toward his mother and old girlfriend, which robbed him of intimacy with everyone in his life including his wife. Edward needed to forgive his mother for leaving a quarter of a century ago. He also needed to let go of the things in his life over which he had limited or no control—his wife's behavior and his daughter's health. Certainly, Edward could make good and rational decisions for his and his family's well-being, but this would not guarantee that they would live long and satisfying lives. To release what wasn't his to own made sense to Edward, even if he did become acutely aware of a temporary increase in his feeling of vulnerability when he admitted his powerlessness.

Edward wrote a letter to release his resentment of his mother and to consider whether he wanted to establish a better relationship now. He elected to release the anger but maintain a distance between them. He liked the idea of improving intimacy with his wife and daughter by reinvesting the energy that he would have spent worrying about them into family time and acts of kindness and generosity toward them.

Your Turn: Use the Truths to Help Laurie

Laurie is a 36-year-old corporate executive. She is happily married and is the proud parent of two pre-teen children. Despite her personal and professional accomplishments, she struggles with making decisions. Though successful in the business world, she frequently questions herself. She graduated in the top five of her high school class but never felt that she was good enough. In talking about her life, she admits that her mother has been overly involved with her life, her decisions, her relationships, and her parenting. Laurie has always wanted her mother's approval. Accordingly, she pushed herself to excel in school and business, but her mother's hypercritical nature always leaves her feeling disappointed and discouraged. Her mother struggled with alcoholism for years, used excessive physical punishment, and blamed Laurie for many family issues. Whenever Laurie expressed her own thoughts, her mother rejected her and overreacted. Recently Laurie has been consumed by negative thoughts about herself, which interfere with work and cause many sleepless nights. She has also become more angry with her mother and short-tempered with her children, especially when they disagree with her. Laurie is struggling with using alcohol to deal with her emotions and entertaining thoughts of having an affair with a coworker whom she flirts with for his attention and approval.

Now use what you've learned to help Laurie deal with her uncertainty, anger, alcohol abuse, and impending infidelity. Go through each of the truths and, using the questions provided as guidance, think of others Laurie might ask herself and reflect on.

Truth #1: Emotions are not mysterious visitors; they can be identified and understood.

- ▶ Why have you become angry at your kids? Are they suddenly behaving a lot worse than in the past or are you angry about something else?

- ▶ When you were growing up, what were you most angry about? Do certain situations still trigger your anger?

- ▶ Do you see any commonalities in the behaviors of your mother and your children that make you angry? Do they say or do similar things that make you feel like you're not in control or that they're criticizing you in some way?

- ▶ Are your reactions more a statement about you and less about your kids?

Truth #2: You can change your compulsive behaviors if you change your thoughts and address your feelings.

▶ What contributes to your feeling so indecisive and uncertain when you've achieved so much in your life?

▶ When you struggle with a decision, what thoughts run through your head? When you take a step and analyze these thoughts, do they seem valid? Or are they reflex thoughts, things you've told yourself all your life?

▶ How might you change your thoughts in these situations to reflect a more realistic outlook?

▶ Have you considered using cognitive restructuring to catch yourself when negative self-statements begin and replace them with positive, constructive statements grounded in reality?

Truth #3: Every behavior has an underlying purpose, and it's not always what we think.

▶ What contributes to your recent increase in drinking?

▶ Why do you struggle chronically with making decisions?

▶ What factors contribute to your anger with your family?

▶ When you consider your drinking, indecisiveness, and anger, can you come up with an explanation for all three beyond situational explanations?

Truth #4: We all sabotage ourselves unless we confront our internal saboteur.

▶ Why are you risking your marriage for an affair with your work colleague?

▶ Is it that this work colleague is your "one true love and that you feel you're meant to be with him rather than your husband?" Or are you driven to have an affair for some other reason?

▶ Is it possible that having an affair would make your life less satisfying and lead to more problems than you currently have?

Truth #5: All behavior requires permission so we must learn what we're permitting ourselves to do.

- ► When you were growing up, how did your mother affect your mood? Did you permit her criticism and disapproval to make you feel inadequate? Do you permit her to determine your emotional state?

- ► As an adult, do you give yourself permission to drink to excess? Have you ever tried refusing yourself permission to have more than one drink per night?

- ► Do you permit yourself to cheat on your spouse? Have you told yourself that it's okay for you to have an affair?

Truth #6: Emotional energy is finite and needs to be invested rather than wasted on wishing, worrying, and whining.

- ► During the sleepless nights when you worry constantly, do you feel emotionally exhausted the next day? Is it difficult to accomplish much the next day?

- ► Have you been able to deepen your bonds with your husband or your children since you started worrying all the time and focusing on the negative?

- ► Do you feel that you spend a significant amount of your emotional energy on fantasizing about your coworker? Do you spend more time and energy on that than on thinking about being with your husband?

Truth #7: Our relationships depend on self-empowerment and not on enabling others.

- ► If you had to assign a percentage to the power you've given your mother over how you feel about yourself, what would it be? 10 percent? 25 percent? More?

- ► Who are the people you try most to control? Among your husband, children, mother, and work colleagues, how do you try to change them to make them who you want them to be?

- ► How successful are your efforts to control and change people?

Truth #8: Ego boundaries protect us from rejection, insult, and intimidation.

▶ Did you ever try to protect yourself from your mother's criticisms when you were younger? How do you protect yourself now?

▶ When someone says something negative to you at work, or your kids or spouse do something that upsets you, are you able to step back and recognize that their words and behaviors are about them and not you?

▶ Have you set up any boundaries in your life to protect you from the words and deeds of others? If you were to set them up, what might they protect you from?

Truth #9: You can trust people to be who they are, not who you want them to be.

▶ Do you keep hoping that your mother will become less critical and more tolerant? Do you keep trusting that, after all these years, she will suddenly recognize that she should be more appreciative of who you are?

▶ Do you keep wishing to yourself that your husband would be more dynamic and assertive? Do you keep thinking that your highly energetic and restless son will turn into a quiet, respectful, and serious student?

Truth #10: Time doesn't heal all pain; we heal ourselves by learning how to let go.

▶ What past traumatic event or repeated pattern of negative behaviors still occupies your thoughts? Do you still revisit your mother's critical behaviors and her leaving your family when you were young? Are the feelings associated with your mother's actions and attitudes bottled up inside?

▶ Do you make an effort to remember and express these feelings to your spouse, a close friend, or a therapist?

▶ Do you feel these feelings deeply—so deeply that evoke a strong reaction, such as tears?

▶ Have you made an effort to release the feelings that hurt so much and to forgive your mother for how she acted?

▶ Have you changed your thinking about your mother? Have you made an effort to stop blaming her for how you are? Have you resolved to reconnect with her in a more emotionally healthy way?

Your Personal Truths

Now it's simply a question of putting together everything you've learned in this book and applying it to whatever problems or issues you're concerned about. We don't want to make this sound easy, but it's not particularly difficult either, once you get the hang of it. Getting the hang of it involves familiarizing yourself with the 10 Truths, being aware of them as you go through your daily life, and applying them in various situations. The exercises found at the end of each chapter were designed to help you get some of this practice. Here's a final exercise that will help you maintain a Truths exercise regimen.

❑ Truth #1: Try to identify an emotion that overcomes you without any discernible cause. It can be sadness, shame, or whatever feeling surfaces frequently. Write the word describing this emotion on a piece of paper, and then draw arrows away from it to five to 10 possible precipitating events. It can be a specific situation (for example, your significant other was rude to you) or it can be a more general cause (for example, free-floating frustration from never having time to yourself). Use these causes as clues to investigate why you feel the way you do.

❑ Truth #2: Focus on the thoughts and feelings that accompany and seem to precipitate your compulsive behaviors and create a change strategy. Write a "before" and "after" statement—your thoughts and feelings before you were aware of this Truth, and how you want to change your thoughts and feelings now. Use the contrast to keep reminding yourself how certain thoughts and feelings reinforce your compulsive behaviors, and how others take you away from them.

❑ Truth #3: Analyze your most mystifying behavior—a behavior that seemingly is counterproductive yet you engage in it repeatedly. Try and dig deep to discover what you get out of it. Is it a ritual that makes you feel good? Is it a way for you to rebel? To analyze this behavior, go beyond the surface reason you engage in it. If it helps, force yourself to go down three levels. For instance: at Level 1, I smoke because it makes me feel good; at Level 2, I feel good because smoking relaxes me and take away my anxiety; and at Level 3, I feel less anxious because smoking makes me feel cool and in control, and I typically don't feel this way.

❑ Truth #4: Create a "word portrait" of your internal saboteur by describing when it is likely to emerge and act against your best interests; what it is likely to encourage you to do or say; how you rationalize its actions; and what outcomes please it. Think about the times that you have talked yourself out of a goal. Identify negative self-statements. Determine what your saboteur is protecting you from.

❑ Truth #5: Create a list of your negative permissions (things you allow yourself to do that have negative consequences) in the following areas: romantic relationships, family, work, addictions. Make the list concise and precise. For instance, "I permit myself to criticize my wife" or "I allow myself to drink and drive." Identify your internal justifications, rationalizations, intellectualizations, and other excuses that allow you to choose behaviors that are inappropriate or destructive.

❑ Truth #6: Reinvest your emotional energy. On any given day, keep a small notebook handy and make a check mark every time you find yourself wishing something were different than it is, worrying about something that you have no control over, or whining about your particular situation. Use all the check marks on the page as a reminder and motivation to stop wishing, worrying, and whining and devote more of your emotional energy to things you're truly passionate about—your spouse, your family, your job, and so on.

Rather than complaining about something outside of your control, choose to pursue a goal, hold yourself accountable, be a role model, set your standards high, and live up to them.

❑ Truth #7: Identify the one person in your life who has the greatest impact on your mood. Make a conscious effort to take power away from this person and reclaim that power for yourself. On a daily basis, repeat to yourself: "[person's name] cannot, should not, and will not determine if I'm happy, sad, or mad." Remind yourself that your happiness should not be dependent on someone else's dysfunction. Don't expect someone to behave differently than their history.

❑ Truth #8: Draw your boundaries—literally. On a piece of paper, write "me" and then around it draw lines and write on the other side of these lines simple descriptions of who usually rejects, insults, and intimidates you. For instance: "[significant other's name] insults how I look" or "[boss's name] threatens to give me a bad review." This drawing should serve as a reminder that what they do reflects on them, not you.

❑ Truth #9: Redefine your expectations for the person in your life who most frequently disappoints you. Recreate these expectations based on this person's behavioral history. Tell yourself that how he/she has behaved in the past is the way he/she is most likely to behave in the future. Recognize that whatever traits and tendencies this person displayed before, he/she is likely to display again.

❑ Truth #10: Find a trusted friend or therapist to help you take the five steps of letting go: remembering, feeling, expressing, releasing, and changing thinking. Refuse to be passive and expect time to help you get better. Take an active role in your emotional health.

The Truth Hurts, Helps, and Heals

Just as time doesn't heal all wounds, these Truths are not a panacea. They're not magically going to cure you of your addictions, lift your depression overnight, or transform you from a failure to a success in 10 easy steps. What they will do, however, is provide you with insights about yourself that will make a huge, albeit gradual, difference in all areas of your life.

Understanding how your mind works is essential. As you learn why you think, feel and act the way you do, you gain greater awareness of who you are. This awareness translates into greater control. The mind is like any sophisticated tool; the more you understand its functions and fallibilities, the better you will be to use it effectively.

We've written this book to help people use their minds more effectively. As psychologists, we've learned how our patients don't always understand their psychological issues and capabilities, so they get themselves in trouble or they don't use their minds in ways that help them avoid trouble and/or capitalize on opportunities. Through months or even years of therapy, they learn how to know themselves better and live fuller, more meaningful lives.

This book isn't a substitute for therapy, but for many people with less serious emotional issues, it is exactly what is needed. Possessing the 10 Truths is like owning a manual for the mind. It will provide you with directions for dealing with most of the situations life throws at you, and it will give you the knowledge to handle these challenges well. As you close this book and go out into the world, we have one final piece of advice: Let the 10 Truths be your guide.

Bibliography

Allport, Gordon. *Theories of Personality*. New York: John Wiley and Sons, 1978.

Bandura, Albert. *Self-efficacy: The exercise of control*. New York: Freeman, 1997.

———. "Self efficacy: toward a unifying theory of behavioral change." *Psychological Review* 84 (1977): 191–215.

The Big Book of Alcoholics Anonymous. Alcoholics Anonymous World Services, Inc. 2001.

Berk, Sally Ann. *The Big Little Book of Jewish Wit and Wisdom*. New York: Black Dog and Leventhal Publishers, Inc., 2000.

Bishoff, Steve, and John Wooden. *An American Treasure*. Nashville: Cumberland House Publishing, Inc., 2004.

"Blind Monks Examining an Elephant." en.wikipedia.org/wiki/Blind-men-and-an-Elephant. Accessed August 29, 2006.

Buscaglia, Leo. *Living, Loving, and Learning*. New York: Fawcett Books, 1982.

Cable, Janice. "Our Cheatin' Hearts: Infidelity—How to Stop Before You Start." *Industry Magazine,* August/September (2005): 35.

Cromie, William J. "Anger Can Break Your Heart." *Harvard University Gazette* (September 2006): 21.

Dingfelder, S. "Insincere Apologies Work as Well as Heartfelt Ones." *Monitor on Psychology* 38, (June 2007): 10.

Dinkmeyer, Don C. et. al. *Adlerian Counseling and Psychotherapy*. New York: Wadsworth Publishing Company, Inc., 1979.

Dossey, Larry. *Healing Words: The Power of Prayer and the Practice of Medicine*. San Francisco: Harper and Sons, 1993.

Edwin, David. Clinical Seminar. Johns Hopkins University, Department of Psychiatry and Behavioral Medicine, 1999.

Fay, Jim, and David Funk. *Teaching with Love and Logic: Taking Control of the Classroom*. Golden, Colo: The Love and Logic Press, 1995.

Feldman, Robert. "Why We Lie." *Journal of Basic and Applied Psychology*. AOL Research and Learn (March 15, 2006).

Forward, Susan, and Beckwith, Craig. *Toxic Parents: Overcoming Their Hurtful Legacy and Reclaiming Your Life*. New York: Bantam Books, 1989.

Fredrickson, Barbara, "Cultivating Positive Emotions to Optimize Health and Wellbeing." American Psychological Association Lecture. Quoted in *Prevention and Treatment* 3, (March 7 2000): 64.

Fredrickson, Renee. "Treatment of Survivors of Sexual Abuse." Lecture. Tampa, Fla. 1992.

Gosling, Sam. "Mixed Signals." *Psychology Today* (September/October 2009): 64.

Jeffers, Susan. *Feel the Fear and Do It Anyway*. New York: Fawcett Books, 1987.

Kalb, Claudia. "The Therapist as Scientist." *Newsweek* 27 (March 2006): 51.

Kaplan, Basha and Gail Prince. *Soul Dating to Soul Mating: On the Path Toward Spiritual Partnership*. New York: The Berkeley Publishing Group, 1999.

Langreth, Robert. "Patient Fix Thyself." *Forbes* 9 (April 2007): 80.

Leahy, Robert. *The Worry Cure: Seven Steps to Stop Worry from Stopping You*. New York: Harmony Books, 2005.

Lidz, Franz. "Mickey Gives Him the Slip." *Sports Illustrated* 17 (April 1989): 20.

Lieberman, Matthew. "Taking the Pain Away." *Science* 302 (October 2006): 35.

McHugh, Paul, MD. Clinical Seminar. Johns Hopkins University, Department of Psychiatry and Behavioral Medicine, 1998.

McKay, Kevin M. et. al. "Towards a Feminist Empowerment Model of Forgiveness Psychotherapy." *Psychotherapy: Theory, Research, Practice, Training* 44 (2007), 14–29.

Miller, Michael. "Forgiveness." Harvard Mental Health Letter, December 2004, 6.

———. "How Not to Be Happy." Harvard Mental Health Letter. March 2004, 6.

National Household Survey on Drug Abuse, 1993.

"One Day at a Time in Al-Anon." New York: Al-Anon Family Group Headquarters, Inc., 1989.

Peale, Norman Vincent. *The Power of Positive Thinking*. New York: Fireside, 2003.

Peck, M. Scott. *The Road Less Traveled*. New York: Simon and Schuster, 1978.

Powers, M.B., et al. "Disentangling the Effects of Safety-Behavior Utilization and Safety-Behavior Availability During Exposure-Based Treatment: A Placebo-Controlled Trial." *Journal of Consulting and Clinical Psychology* Vol. 72, No. 3 (May–June 2004): 448–54.

Prochaska, James O., and C. C. DiClemente. "Stages and Processes of Self-Change of Smoking: Toward an Integrative Model of Change." *Journal of Consulting and Clinical Psychology* 51 (1983): 390–395.

Ruben, Ann. Lecture. Florida Psychological Association, 2007.

Scott, Walter. "Personality Parade." *Parade Magazine*, 10 (June 2007): 2.

Seligman, Martin. *Learned Optimism*. New York: Pocket Books, 1990.

———. *Authentic Happiness: Using the New Positive Psychology to Realize Your Potential for Lasting Fulfillment*. New York: The Free Press, 2002.

Shakespeare, William. *Hamlet. The Complete Works of William Shakespeare*. Edited by Hardin Craig. Chicago: Scott, Foresman and Company, 1961.

Shenk, Joshua. "What Makes Us Happy?" *The Atlantic* (June 2009): 48.

Simon, Syd, and Suzanne Simon. "Healing From Emotional Hurt." Lecture. Holiday Inn, Clearwater, Fla. 1987.

Underwood, Marion. "Social Aggression Among Girls." *Monitor on Psychology* (2003): 64.

Weingarten, Abby. "Impassioned Responses." *Herald Tribune*, 4 March 2004, 4E.

"Where Are They Now? No Longer Busts." *Sports Illustrated* (July 12 2004).

Index

A

Act, 91
acting compulsively, 11
acting in an irrational or confusion
      way, 11
Action, 137
Adapt, 90
Address, 89
Al-Anon, 131
Alice, Kathryn, 145

anger, 27-28
anxiety, 23-24
artistic expression, 187-188
avoidance and short-term benefits,
      65-66

B

Barr, Roseanne, 161
behavior and the underlying
      purpose, 9
behavior as a problem, 103

value of what you learn, maximize the, 12-13

worrying, 11
worrying, chronic, 70-72

About the Authors

Dr. Harold E. Shinitzky is in private practice in Clearwater, St. Petersburg, and Tierra Verde, Florida. He currently consults for several counties, states, and countries as well as for public and independent schools in the development, implementation, and evaluation of adolescent prevention initiatives. He is also the national consultant to the Police Athletic Leagues, and the consulting sports psychologist for Athlete Connections, an educational life skills program helping student-athletes transition to life after sports. His specialties include sports psychology and child psychology.

Dr. Shinitzky has published articles on the topics of substance abuse prevention programs for youth as well as on the topic of provider-patient interview and communication skills training. Dr. Shinitzky is a founding member of AbleVillage.com, a Web portal for children and adults with disabilities. He has been the mental health correspondent for Radio Disney and Fox television in Tampa, and for "Fast Forward" on ABC in Baltimore, Maryland.

Dr. Shinitzky is the former director of the Assessment/Intervention Team (AIT) Prevention Services at the Johns Hopkins University School of Medicine, Department of Pediatrics. In this capacity, Dr. Shinitzky developed and facilitated after-school peer-oriented prevention groups for high-risk youth.

Dr. Shinitzky is the recipient of the 2009 Florida Psychological Association Distinguished Psychologist award, and the 2009 Florida Psychological Association Outstanding Contributions to Psychology in the Public Interest award. Dr. Shinitzky was selected as the recipient of the Martin Luther King, Jr. Award for Community Service in 2000. He received the Distinguished Faculty, Excellence in Teaching award from Towson University, Department of Psychology Psi Chi Chapter in 1997 and 1999, as well as the Most Helpful Doc award from the pediatric residents at the Johns Hopkins University School of Medicine. He was also included in the Who's Who in America of 2003.

Dr. Shinitzky has presented internationally and nationally to major mental health organizations and medical societies on the topic of "best practice" models in the prevention of high-risk youth. He presented to the sixth annual United Nations International Conference on Substance Abuse in Italy, and recently presented to the Drug Prevention Networks of the Americas in Buenos Aires, Argentina.

Dr. Shinitzky is on the national advisory boards of Drug Free America, The Learning Partnership, and the Applied Institute of Forensic Psychology. He also served as a member of the committee on women and minorities at the Johns Hopkins University. He was a Robert Wood Johnson Join Together national fellow, as well as a fellow of the Center for Substance Abuse Prevention, Faculty Development Project. Previously, he was president of the Baltimore Psychological Association. Dr. Shinitzky was recently appointed to the Medical Advisory Board for the Florida Office of Drug Control, and has been elected by his peers for a fourth consecutive term as president of the Florida Psychological Association, Pinellas Chapter.

Dr. Christopher Cortman has treated patients with a wide range of issues in the 50,000 hours of psychotherapy he has facilitated: relationships, anxiety, depression, and grief. He has a sub-specialty treating the highly traumatized: war veterans, rape victims, and abuse and cult survivors. In addition, Dr. Cortman has served as a consulting psychologist to Mediplex, a hospital for brain-injured patients, and was the director of Allied Health Practitioners at Sarasota Palms Hospital. He was also president of the Lower West Coast chapter of the Florida Psychological Association; director of Gulf Area Psychiatric Services in Venice; consulting psychologist for the Genesis Program, a 28-day residential program for addictions; and consulting psychologist for The Rehabilitation Institute of Sarasota. He's also served as an expert witness for the state of Florida. Currently he is on medical staff at the Venice Regional Medical Center.